Education in a Competitive and Globalizing World

Knowledge Transfer

Practices, Types and Challenges

Education in a Competitive and Globalizing World

Additional books in this series can be found on Nova's website under the Series tab.

Additional e-books in this series can be found on Nova's website under the e-book tab.

Public Health in the 21st Century

Additional books in this series can be found on Nova's website under the Series tab.

Additional e-books in this series can be found on Nova's website under the e-book tab.

EDUCATION IN A COMPETITIVE AND GLOBALIZING WORLD

KNOWLEDGE TRANSFER

PRACTICES, TYPES AND CHALLENGES

DRAGAN ILIC
EDITOR

Nova Science Publishers, Inc.
New York

Library of Congress Cataloging-in-Publication Data

ISBN: 978-1-62081-538-0

Published by Nova Science Publishers, Inc. † New York

Contents

PREFACE

The discipline of knowledge transfer has existed for many years across disciplines, but has more recently gained exposure within the health care field including medicine, nursing, health sciences, public health and health services research. Knowledge transfer is a complex iterative process that aims to implement high quality evidence into practice ensuring that better health outcomes are achieved across different levels including patients, health professionals, health systems and policy makers. This book provides an introduction to the field of knowledge transfer, examining the different approaches to knowledge transfer as well as detailing challenges to its implementation in practice. This book examines what knowledge transfer is, and how it may differ across different contexts and settings.

Chapter 1 - Knowledge transfer aims to close the gap between evidence and practice. It aims to identify and implement knowledge into practice in a timely manner to ensure that optimal outcomes are met. The methods to close the 'evidence to practice' gap form the framework for knowledge transfer. In order to bridge this gap, acknowledge transfer framework needs to identify information gaps, create new knowledge (or obtain existing knowledge), effectively implement it into the relevant setting and evaluate its effectiveness. This chapter will provide a commentary defining the concept of knowledge transfer and outline the development of the DIER knowledge transfer framework.

Chapter 2 - Alliances as a form of inter-organizational cooperation are increasing in number and importance on the global business scale, and numerous reasons can be given to explain this. Among other benefits that alliances can bring to those who create them, organizational learning and knowledge transfer have become particularly important. Alliances are used as a means of achieving both single and double loop learning, for exploration as well as for the exploitation purposes, and are thought to be particularly powerful in tacit knowledge transfer. Theoretical review in this chapter addresses: first, the issues of knowledge transfer and organizational learning in strategic alliances, next, it identifies potential research gaps and finally, it gives propositions that might help future research in this field.

Chapter 3 - Knowledge brokers such as health care professionals and consumer group peer support leaders experience many challenges in transferring and exchanging knowledge for persons with chronic pain and those with work injuries. Meeting the needs of end users and their preferences for considering and integrating knowledge into decision making is not easy. This chapter will provide an overview of the barriers to KT and offer strategies to facilitate ways to meet the needs of end users such as persons with chronic pain that is also sensitive to the contextual and social cultural expectations of the end users. Readers will be introduced to an Interactive Knowledge Transfer Process that can enable formal and informal knowledge brokers to create spaces and opportunities for practical knowledge exchange of research, procedural and health information needed to manage daily and work activities while living with pain. This chapter will also have a focus on what knowledge brokers need to know to help end users successfully appraise information available on the internet.

Chapter 4 - The principles of evidence based practice focus on providing users with the skills to identify, evaluate and implement evidence within a clinical setting. A similar process is also apparent with knowledge transfer, which also takes into account barriers and facilitators of evidence uptake by stakeholders. This chapter will explore how the principles of evidence based practice may be utilized by individuals to facilitate knowledge transfer from a user's perspective.

Chapter 5 - When a statistical model is designed in a prediction purpose, a major assumption is the absence of evolution in the modeled phenomenon between the training and the prediction stages. Thus, training and future data must be in the same feature space and must have the same distribution. Unfortunately, this assumption turns out to be often false in real-world applications. For instance, biological motivations could lead to classify individuals from a given species when only individuals from another species are available for training. In regression, we would sometimes use a predictive model for data having not exactly the same distribution that the training data used for estimating the model. This chapter presents techniques for transfering a statistical model estimated from a source population to a target population. Three tasks of statistical learning are considered: Probabilistic classification (parametric and semi-parametric), linear regression (includingmixture of regressions) and model-based clustering (Gaussian and Student). In each situation, the knowledge transfer is carried out by introducing parametric links between both populations. The use of such transfer techniques would improve the performance of learning by avoiding much expensive data labeling efforts.

Chapter 6 - The biotechnology industry is characterized by a high intensity in knowledge creation and innovation. Biotechnology companies are constantly affected by knowledge flows so this industry is an interesting field to study knowledge transfer strategies. In this chapter the authors analyze the knowledge transfer strategies of three Spanish biotechnology companies, PharmaMar, Neocodex and Digna Biotech. With this aim an exploratory case study was carried out by the authors, which is based on the model of technological knowledge transfer developed by Bozeman (2000). The results of this study provide a comprehensive overview of the aspects that characterize different ways to understand a knowledge transfer strategy and the results that are obtained from its application.

Chapter 7 - Poster presentations are a common-place feature of many modern academic and professional settings. Based upon the wide range of professional groups that utilise the medium and the multitude of local, national and international meetings at which they are presented, it may be fair to estimate that millions are undertaken every year. As a stand-alone medium however, they are not best suited to facilitate knowledge transfer. This chapter looks at how we can make the most of the many opportunities for poster presentation and use facilitated dialogue to increase the potential to communicate our findings, opinions and research to others. In particular, it considers those aspects of knowledge transfer commonly found in both the business and conference setting; namely the concepts of knowledge / research dissemination and its subsequent utilization by the receiver. In considering these aspects, this chapter looks to demonstrate that although the academic poster is a favoured medium of visualising knowledge, there are further considerations to be made, if we are to effectively transfer that knowledge to others.

Chapter 8 - This chapter is a practical guide to developing an evidence based guideline (EBG). It begins with a discussion about EBGs, their place within health information overall, why they are important and why it is important that they are developed in a rigorous and systematic way. While EBG development guidance is available, there is inconsistency in the amount of detail across this guidance and it has been suggested that practical information to complement existing resources may be helpful. Therefore, logistics of EBG development and practical step by step information about their development is discussed using an example of a nationally approved EBG in the area of polycystic ovary syndrome (PCOS). The authors also provide directions to other helpful resources, tools and templates for each step. Practical concepts covered include establishing a multidisciplinary evidence based guideline development group (EBGDG); clinical question development and prioritisation; evidence review and synthesis; drafting of recommendations; obtaining consensus among the EBGDG; and preparing and finalising the EBG for dissemination.

Chapter 9 - Effective knowledge transfer between researchers, educators, and clinicians is essential for maintaining best practice in the health disciplines. It is the method by which we aim to enhance the health service delivery for our communities. This chapter examines methods of knowledge transfer for supporting health professional clinical performance. Competent clinical skills are a combination of theoretical knowledge, manual handling, and effective communication, encapsulated in the clinician-client interaction. Training for optimum performance of clinical skills is a complex and enduring task. Health professional education is a continuum, beginning from entry into an undergraduate program, and continues until the health professional leaves their chosen discipline. This chapter focuses on innovative methods utilised within an undergraduate clinical skills program, techniques for supporting transfer of knowledge to a clinical environment, and the continuing education of health professionals. It tackles issues relating to access and utilisation of educational technologies, and facilitation of a successful knowledge transfer culture.

Chapter 10 - Journal clubs have been operating in various formats for over 100 years in the medical field. Journal clubs aim to promote effective knowledge transfer of medical evidence to clinicians and subsequent uptake into the clinical setting. Clinician awareness, agreement, adoption and adherence of evidence may all act as barriers when translating high quality evidence into practice. This chapter will provide a commentary on the use of journal clubs in knowledge transfer and also proposes a method of utilizing journal clubs as complex interventions as a strategy to translate evidence into practice effectively.

In: Knowledge Transfer: Practices, Types and Challenges
Editor: Dragan Ilic
ISBN: 978-1-62081-538-0

Chapter 1

WHAT IS KNOWLEDGE TRANSFER?

Dragan Ilic*
Department of Epidemiology and Preventive Medicine,
School of Public Health and Preventive Medicine,
Monash University, VIC, Australia

ABSTRACT

Knowledge transfer aims to close the gap between evidence and practice. It aims to identify and implement knowledge into practice in a timely manner to ensure that optimal outcomes are met. The methods to close the 'evidence to practice' gap form the framework for knowledge transfer. In order to bridge this gap, acknowledge transfer framework needs to identify information gaps, create new knowledge (or obtain existing knowledge), effectively implement it into the relevant setting and evaluate its effectiveness. This chapter will provide a commentary defining the concept of knowledge transfer and outline the development of the DIER knowledge transfer framework.

INTRODUCTION

James Lind was a Scottish physician, who in 1747 conducted the first clinical trial to investigate the hypothesis that the consumption of citrus fruits could cure scurvy. [1]. As a surgeon on the *HMS Salisbury*, Dr Lind hypothesized that the lack of Vitamin C intake by sailors, due to the lack of suitable food on board the ship for the period of time, was directly linked to the increased outbreak of scurvy on board the *HMS Salisbury*. To answer this clinical question, Dr Lind divided 12 sailors into six groups. Each of the sailors received the same diet, but each group were supplemented with; cider, sulphuric acid, vinegar, seawater, oranges and lemons, and barley water. After approximately one-week of treatment, only the sailors allocated to receiving oranges and lemons were fit for duty. In 1753 Dr Lind published these results; however the findings were not translated into practice until 1795.

* Corresponding author: E-mail: dragan.ilic@monash.edu

The case of Dr James Lind was an early case of how knowledge transferworks. Dr Lin was presented with an information gap, new knowledge is created (or existing knowledge is collated if possible), with findings implemented into practice with the aim of changing behaviour and improving outcomes. However, knowledge transfer is not always an easy process – with a number of potential obstacles hindering uptake of evidence into practice. A variety of factors may influence why high quality evidence is not implemented in practice [2]. Subsequently, many users, and patients within the healthcare system, will receive ineffectual care. This inefficient care has the potential to place great strain on the healthcare system.

This chapter will provide a commentary defining the concept of knowledge transfer and introduce the DIER knowledge transfer framework. It will provide an overview of the various steps associated with this knowledge transfer framework, and how it may be effectively implemented across various settings.

What is Knowledge Transfer?

Knowledge transfer is a term that has existed for many years, but more recently gained great prominence across a variety of health disciplines including public health, medicine, nursing and allied health. [3]Knowledge transfer aims to close the information gap between evidence, be it existing or newly created, and practice.

Table I. Definition of terms relating to knowledge transfer

Term	Definition
Knowledge transfer	A term used in healthcare, as well as fields outside of healthcare. The focus is on providing all relevant stakeholders with high quality evidence (usually research based).
Knowledge translation	Similar to knowledge transfer, with the focus on addressing the gap between knowledge, and the implementation of this knowledge by stakeholders.
Knowledge exchange	Highlights the differences in organisational culture, which may act as barriers to the implementation of knowledge in practice. Knowledge exchange brings together researchers and users in an attempt to override barriers, and promote knowledge exchange to the stakeholders and end-users.
Research utilisation	A term that has been entrenched in the nursing field. Research utilisation focuses on moving research findings into practice within the appropriate clinical setting.
Implementation science	Implementation science has a greater focus on the methods used to promote the uptake of research findings into practice.

* Adapted from Graham et al. [2].

This information is then implemented, via any form of tailored intervention, to the target audience in a timely manner to ensure optimal uptake of services or products. The methods used to facilitate this process can generally be defined as 'knowledge transfer'. [3]

One of the confusing issues within the field of knowledge transfer is the terminology associated with the discipline itself. Table 1 illustrates the variety of terms that have been used to define knowledge transfer. Whilst all of those terms are grounded in the definition of knowledge transfer, certain differences should be noted. Translational research focusses on the transfer of basic science into clinical applications – the 'bench to bedside' phenomenon. [2]. It should also be noted that any continuing education or continuing professional development interpretations should not be confused with knowledge transfer – since these formats focus on the increasing individual competence rather than a broader spectrum that includes a wide range of stakeholders. [2]

Why is Knowledge Transfer Important?

In healthcare a verse from the Hippocratic Oath read, *'I will prescribe regimens for the good of my patients according to my ability and my judgment and never do harm to anyone'*. Whilst it may seem that this would common sense, the implications of failing to use research evidence to inform decision making are still apparent.

The case of Dr James Lind probably was not the first, and not the last, time that research evidence has not reached users in'reasonable' time. In 1946 Dr Benjamin Spock, an American pediatrician, first published his book entitled, *'Baby and child care'*, which provided advise for parents on how to care for their babies, infants and children. By 1998 it is estimated that the book sold in excess of 50,000,000 copies worldwide. During that period, all editions of the book recommended that 'babies should be put to sleep on their fronts…'.[4]In his book, Dr Spock reasoned that this approach would reduce the risk of infants choking on their own vomit. However, research evidence from the 1970s suggested that this practice may be harmful, and be linked to sudden infant death syndrome (SIDS). Furthermore, it was not until the late 1980s and early 1990s that the advice was revised, with parents advised to put their babies to sleep on their back. During this time it is estimated that over 50,000 babies worldwide died from SIDS.

In Australia during the 1980s researchers identified that maternal dietary and supplemental folate intake around the time of conception protects against neural tube defects (NTDs). [5]Subsequent studies also confirmed up to 70% protective effect. However, it was not until 1992 that dedicated health promotion activities were implemented, which resulted in an increase of 30% in women taking folate, and 29% fall in NTDs. [6, 7] Conversely, there examples where evidence that indicates that a particular treatment is not beneficial still gets consumed due to habit. For example, evidence from systematic reviews has identified benefit of consuming Vitamin C for preventing and treating the common cold. [8]Despite this evidence, a large international demand for Vitamin C remains from the public, who still believe in a beneficial effect through its consumption.

Such cases have promoted a greater emphasis on knowledge transfer in healthcare to change user (clinicians, patient and policy maker) behaviour. However, changing behaviour is not a simple process. It involves the evaluation of the entire organizational structure, with specific intervention tailored to various stakeholders in a bid to change behaviour. [9]

The DIER Knowledge Transfer Framework

A variety of knowledge transfer models have been created. [2, 3, 9-11]The DIER knowledge transfer framework builds on these existing models but also places an emphasis on the knowledge transfer process being iterative in nature. Figure 1 illustrates the DIER knowledge transfer framework, with a description of each step as follows;

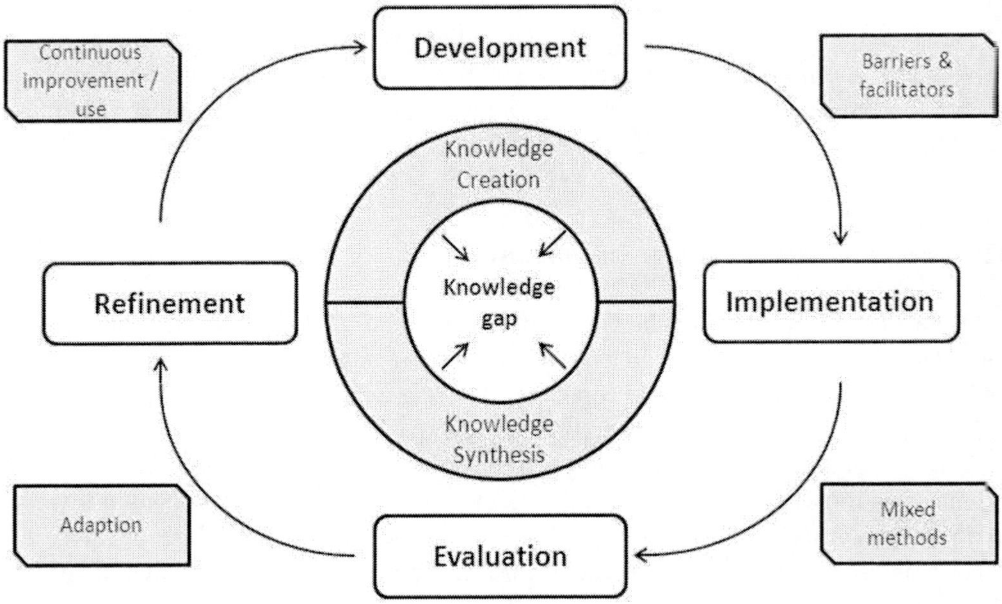

Figure 1. The DIER knowledge transfer framework.

Knowledge Gap

The DIER knowledge transfer framework begins with the knowledge, or information, gap. It is this knowledge gap that will facilitate the DIER knowledge transfer process. The knowledge gap may be answered either by the creation of new knowledge (through new research findings), or the synthesis of existing knowledge from original studies, systematic reviews (and likewise synthesis) or other third party synopses and appraisals. [3]It is important to note that in some circumstances there will not be sufficient evidence to answer the knowledge gap.

This type of 'information' is still useful in the DIER knowledge transfer framework, as it provides useful transfer of information gaps within the evidence to key stakeholders. For example, the issue of screening for prostate cancer generated strong debate within the medical community as there was insufficient evidence from high quality evidence to support, or refute, the merits of screening. [12]

This knowledge was important to transfer to key stakeholders (in this case men, clinicians and policy makers) since there was no evidence to support that screening would decrease the risk of prostate cancer mortality, but also no evidence that it would increase the harms associated with screening (e.g. over-diagnosis).

Effectively transferring this knowledge to stakeholders transformed the manner in which prostate cancer screening was discussed – with shared decision making on the merits of screening discussed between patient and doctor promoted in the absence of solid evidence.

Development

Once the knowledge gap has answered, the intervention that will be used to implement the 'new' knowledge must be developed. In tailoring the intervention, it is essential that all key stakeholders are consulted in order to establish barriers and facilitators to the intervention.

This will permit the intervention to be tailored to meet the needs of the various target audience. Issues such as framing of information, mode of delivery and the timing of the intervention will all impact upon the relative success of the knowledge transfer. For example, clinicians might prefer a 15 minute academic detailing session, which is supplemented by information on a website to facilitate the knowledge transfer due to time commitments.

Conversely, the same information delivered to a policy maker might consist of a full-day workshop. Regardless of how the intervention is delivered across stakeholders, it is essential that the information across all versions remains constant, whilst the intervention itself is adapted to suit the environment in which it will be implemented.

Whilst it is important to consider what type of intervention will most succeed in promoting knowledge transfer, it is also important to understand the cost implications and potential limitations presented. It might well be desirable to develop a multifocal intervention, however practical and cost issues may dictate a more pragmatic intervention.

Implementation

Pilot testing of the intervention is required before its implementation. A key step in the pilot testing of the implementation phase is discussion with key stakeholders about the practical barriers and facilitators to the implementation of the intervention. Key consideration must be given to the different levels to which the intervention will be implemented e.g. individual/team, patient/health professional, clinical/administrative and disciplines (e.g. medicine, nursing, allied health etc.).

Each stakeholder will have different barriers and facilitators that require the intervention be adapted to in order to be implemented within the local context presented.

Evaluation

Once implemented it is important to evaluate the effectiveness of the intervention in promoting the knowledge transfer. Endpoints for evaluation include examining the effectiveness of the implementation strategy for the intervention, monitoring uptake of the knowledge/intervention in practice, examining primary and surrogate outcomes and evaluating stakeholder satisfaction. Any evaluation plan should incorporate a mixed-methods approach, which incorporates both quantitative as well as qualitative methodologies.

Quantitative methodologies may consist of questionnaires, audits and data analysis – whilst qualitative methodologies may include individual interviews, focus group discussions or field observations.

Refinement

Evaluation of the implementation phase will provide useful feedback regarding the effectiveness of the intervention and implementation strategies. The intervention and implementation strategies should be adapted according to the evaluation before the DIER cycle begins again. This refinement phase should be undertaken consistently, even in the event that the original evaluation is positive, in order to ensure continuous improvement, and use of the intervention by the desired stakeholders.

Conclusion

The discipline of knowledge transfer aims to convey knowledge into action, however ensuring that this process is efficient and effective remains challenging. The development of models such as the DIER knowledge transfer framework provides users with a structure on which to draw upon when devising methods of knowledge transfer relative to their specific contexts. Knowledge transfer can facilitate the exchange of knowledge and ideas only when local barriers and facilitators are recognized and adapted to.

References

[1] Tansella M: Implementation of science: understanding the translation of evidence into practice. *British Journal of Psychiatry* 2009, 195:283-285.

[2] Graham I, Logan J, Harrison M, Straus S, Tetroe J, Caswell W, Robinson N: Lost in knowledge translation: time for a map?*The Journal of Continuing Education in the Health Professions* 2006, 26:13-24.

[3] Lang E, Wyer P, Haynes B: Knowledge translation: closing the evidence-to-practice gap. *Annals of Emergency Medicine* 2007, 49:355-363.

[4] Spock B: Baby and Child Care. London: Bodley Head; 1946.

[5] Bower C, Stanley F: Dietary folate as a risk for the neural-tube defects: evidence from a case-control study in Western Australia.*Medical Journal of Australia* 1989, 150: 613-619.

[6] Bower C, Knowles S, Nicol D: Changes in folate supplementation, and in serum and red cell folate levels in antenatal patients over the course of a health promotion project for the prevention of neural tube defects. *Medical Journal of Australia* 1997, 37: 267-271.

[7] Bower C, Blum L, O'Daly K, Higgins C, Loutsky F, Kosky C: Promotion of folate for the prevention of neural tube defects: knowledge of and use of periconceptional folic

acid supplements in Western Australia, 1992-1995. *Australia and New Zealand Journal of Public Health* 1997, 21:716-721.

[8] Hemilä H, Chalker E, Douglas B: Vitamin C for preventing and treating the common cold. *Cochrane Database of Systematic Reviews* 2007, Issue 3:Art. No.: CD000980. DOI: 000910.001002/14651858.CD14000980.pub14651853.

[9] Straus S, Tetroe J, Graham I: Defining knowledge transfer. *CMAJ* 2009, 181:165-168.

[10] Davis D, Evans M, Jadad A, Perrier L, Rath D, Ryan D, Sibbald G, Straus S, Rappolt S, Wowk M *et al*: The case for knowledge translation: shortening the journey from evidence to effect. *BMJ* 2003, 327:33-35.

[11] Pentland D, Forsyth K, Maciver D, Walsh M, Murray R, Irvine L, Sikora S: Key characteristics of knowledge transfer and exchange in healthcare: integrative literature review. *Journal of Advanced Nursing* 2011, 67:1408-1425.

[12] Ilic D, O'Connor D, Green S, Wilt T: Screening for prostate cancer: an updated Cochrane systematic review. *BJU International* 2011, 107:882-891.

In: Knowledge Transfer: Practices, Types and Challenges
Editor: Dragan Ilic
ISBN: 978-1-62081-538-0

Chapter 2

KNOWLEDGE TRANSFER AND ORGANIZATIONAL LEARNING THROUGH STRATEGIC ALLIANCES: THEORETICAL REVIEW AND RESEARCH PERSPECTIVES

Ana Aleksić Mirić*
Faculty of Economics, University of Belgrade, Serbia

ABSTRACT

Alliances as a form of inter-organizational cooperation are increasing in number and importance on the global business scale, and numerous reasons can be given to explain this. Among other benefits that alliances can bring to those who create them, organizational learning and knowledge transfer have become particularly important. Alliances are used as a means of achieving both single and double loop learning, for exploration as well as for the exploitation purposes, and are thought to be particularly powerful in tacit knowledge transfer. Theoretical review in this chapter addresses: first, the issues of knowledge transfer and organizational learning in strategic alliances, next, it identifies potential research gaps and finally, it gives propositions that might help future research in this field.

INTRODUCTION

This chapter addresses the issue of knowledge transfer and organizational learning in strategic alliances. Alliances as a form of inter-organizational cooperation are increasing in number and importance on global business scale, and numerous reasons can be given to explain this. The most common arguments are the following: the possibilities that alliances open for entering the *"forbidden"* and otherwise unavailable market, the expansion of strategic potentials, the share of risks and costs, the availability of rare resources, the increase

* E-mail address: anaa@ekof.bg.ac.rs

in profitability, the decrease in number of competitors; financing capital investments, the exploitation of the existing and the exploration of new findings, as well as maximizing learning possibilities (Inkpen, Ramaswamy, 2006; Osborn, Hagedoorn, 1997; Inkpen, Beamish, 1997; Yashino, Rangan, 1995; Hennart, 1991; Kogut, 1988). The unique logic, underlying this list of goals is that by creating an alliance, a company in fact creates an opportunity to achieve a number of strategically important goals, much faster, with significantly lower costs, and with greater flexibility than it would if it individually pursued business action. Therefore, these goals are not mutually exclusive, but in most cases are mutually supportive.

Contemporary theory and practice recognize organizational learning and transfer of knowledge as one of the main reasons why companies enter strategic alliances today. Alliances are used as a means of achieving both single and double loop learning, for exploration as well as for exploitation purposes. Alliances are thought to be particularly potential in the transfer of tacit knowledge[1]. Even in cases when companies have not initially entered strategic partnership with an intention to learn and increase knowledge depositories, the very environment of cooperation among companies possessing different knowledge and skills, different competencies and ways of applying them in practice, opens new possibilities for learning, gaining knowledge and acquiring new skills (Inkpen, 1998). In the research of organizational learning and knowledge transfer in strategic alliances, several perspectives have emerged as the most distinguished ones. The works of Inkpen, Child, Grant and Baden-Fuller, and Lyles stand out as they give a deep, valid and systematic account of the research done in the area so far, and systematize the basic knowledge on the process of learning within alliances. On the other hand, they point to the main-streams in further research.

Research led by Inkpen has laid the foundations for studying knowledge management processes in strategic alliances (Inkpen, Crossan, 1995; Inkpen, 1996, 1997, 1998; Inkpen, Dinur, 1998, Inkpen, Ramaswamy, 2006). His work affirmed the learning perspective in international interorganizational cooperation. He recognizes the whole complexity of the process of learning through strategic alliances, and demystifies ungrounded platonic understandings by explaining how demanding, frustrating and, more often than not, misunderstood knowledge management in alliances is. He emphasizes that creating a stimulating learning environment within strategic alliance is an exception, rather than a rule. His research relies on the following four processes as key factors enabling the transfer of knowledge in strategic alliances: the share of technology, the interaction between a partner and an alliance, the rotation of employees and strategic integration. A significant corpus of results of Inkpen's research refers to the analysis of the manager's role in the process of learning within strategic alliance, then, to research into the phenomenon of managerial learning, to the share and the integration of managerial knowledge into an organizational context, to institutional learning, and finally to the analysis of the relationship between learning and alliance performances.

Research led by Child (Child, Czeglédy, 1996; Child, Markoczy, 1993; Child, Rodriques, 1996, Child, 2003) gave a deep insight into the nature of learning process in strategic

[1] The distinction between tacit and explicit knowledge can be made by the characteristic of transferability. While explicit knowledge can be easily transferred through communication, tacit knowledge can be transferred only through application and acquired through practice (Grant, 1996:111). Tacit knowledge is embedded within a specific context whereas explicit knowledge is open and easily achievable (Polanyi, 1966; Cummings, 2001: 18).

alliances, managerial behavior, competitive and collaborative aims that partners can have in the context of learning and knowledge transfer, learning during the evolution of alliances and the barriers which can stop or inhibit the learning process. From strategic aspect, these works were among the first to point to the importance of clearly defining the aims of strategic partnership, and they were among the first to show the willingness to use a strategic alliance as an opportunity to learn. From an organizational aspect, Child's research contributed to the affirmation of organizational assumptions for learning, emphasizing the required organizational capacities for learning, organizational ability to accept new knowledge, as well as the ability to handle the process of knowledge acquisition.

The work of Grant and Baden-Fuller (2004) affirmed a knowledge accessing theory of strategic alliances, arguing that alliances can prove to be superior to individual organizations when their aim is to provide the integration of knowledge different in kind. The work led by Lyles is particularly important as it not only focuses on organizational learning, but also exclusively highlights the area of learning in transition countries through various forms of inter-organizational cooperation (alliances, joint ventures etc.). Thorough analysis of the empirical evidence of knowledge management in strategic alliances has been recently given by Meier (2011).

In addition, specific perspectives on organizational learning and knowledge transfer in strategic alliances have been developed as well: technological perspective of learning and knowledge transfer (Mowery et al., 1996; Dierkes et al., 2001: 282; Zander, Kogut, 1995; Galbraith, 1990; Zander, 1991), cultural perspective (Lane, Beamish, 1990; Luo, 1997, Osborn, Hagedoorn, 1997), perspective of trust (Muthusamy, White, 2005), evolution and life-cycle perspective (Faulkner, 1995; Ariño and de la Torre, 1998; Iyer, 2002; Child, 2003), competition perspective (Khanna, Gulati, Nohria, 1994; Hamel, 1991) and the perspective of organizational fit and absorptive capacity (Cohen, Levinthal, 1990; Lorange, Rose, 1991; Szulanski, 1996; Lane, Lubatkin, 1998; Cummings, 2001; Inkpen, Ramaswamy, 2006).

The aim of this paper is to offer a systematic review of the existing knowledge in organizational learning and knowledge transfer in strategic alliances, to identify potential research gaps and to give propositions that might help in the future research of this issue.

STRATEGIC ALLIANCES

Among different kinds of inter-firm network arrangements, strategic alliances have become one of the highly attractive and commonly used ways in which companies provide for their market survival and competitive advantage. There is no generally accepted definition of strategic alliance in relevant literature.

Alliances are defined as voluntary agreements between firms involving exchange, sharing, or co-development of products, technologies, or services (Inkpen, Ramaswamy, 2006:81, Inkpen, Tsang, 2005: 148, Gulati, 1998: 293); then as forms of cooperation between firms for the purpose of improving the partner's ability to achieve their strategic goals (Child, 2003); and as formal agreements between two or more business organizations to pursue a set of private and common goals through sharing resources (e.g. intellectual property, people, capital, organizational capabilities, and physical assets) in contexts involving contesting markets and uncertainty over outcomes (Ariño et al., 2001: 110).

Yashino and Rangan (1995) suggest that there are three conditions which must be met in order to recognize a partnership as strategic alliance: (1) common decision between two or more companies to enter partnership in order to accomplish the desired goals, and still maintain their independence after creating an alliance; (2) the partners' readiness to share both the benefits which come as a result of creating an alliance and the control over the responsibilities related to the functioning of an alliance, (this might be considered to be both the most important characteristic of alliances and the most difficult task to complete); and (3) the partners constant contribution to the accomplishment of one or more strategic goals.

Alliances are often misunderstood as a form of inter-firm collaboration, as they stand between traditional market forms of inter-organizational collaboration on the one hand, and mergers and acquisitions on the other hand. Inkpen and Ramaswamy note that "*last decade or so it has become fashionable to term any inter-firm relationship an alliance…*(even though) *….most inter-firm relationships lack the requisite elements to be termed alliances* (2006:81)". Ariño and de la Torre (1998) explain that "*alliances include all arrangements between independent firms where each contributes certain assets under its control for a common purpose, and which are structured between the extremes of a spot market contract and a merger or acquisition".*

The dominant characteristic of strategic alliances among other forms of inter-organizational linking is the independence of allies after the partnership has been created. Their independence is constant and characterized by the cooperation between partners when it comes sharing expenses, applying the mechanisms of leadership and coordination, which are all the factors contributing to the complexity of controlling an alliance (Inkpen, 2001: 403). However, though being independent, the partners take responsibility both for themselves and their goals, and for their partner's strategic goals, because they are aware of the fact that the success of the alliance depends on mutual effort and cooperation (Inkpen, Ramaswamy, 2006).

Strategic alliances can be classified according to whether they were formed on contract or ownership basis, with or without forming a new entity. Such a division opens a possibility to analyze the real nature of strategic partnerships which involve making a connection which basically means more than a contract-based relation and less than an integration. Ariño and Reuer (2004) point to the importance of the criterion of ownership and the distinction between ownership-based and non-ownership based partnerships, relying on the fact that distinguishing between contract-based and ownership-based strategic alliances makes no real sense, because every partnership implies forming some kind of contract. Strategic alliances can also be classified according to their position in value chain.

The application of this criterion suggests distinguishing between horizontal and vertical forms of strategic alliances. Horizontal alliances are characterized by forming partnerships between companies which belong to the same branch of industry and the same type of business (*Sony-Philips*, for example), while vertical alliances are based on forming partnerships between partners who belong to different parts of value chain and who are linked in the process of input and output (the output of one company in the chain is the input for the others, like *Toshiba-Time Warner*). Since horizontal alliances are created between companies which belong to the same branch of industry and business, such alliances are often referred to as alliances with competitors (Burgers et al., 1993: 420). Literature also suggests that distinction should be made on the basis of the number of partners who form an alliance.

In this sense, there is a difference between the alliances which were created as a result of joining between two partners and those which consist of more than two companies. The necessity of distinguishing between strategic alliances on functional basis, i.e. strategic alliances in marketing, production, research and development and other functional areas, is also often pointed to.

A more specific and more precise definition of the types of strategic alliances is provided by Inkpen (2001: 404), who defines alliances as entities involving industrial consortiums, technical trainings, supplier/buyback arrangements, production/assembly arrangements, patent licensing, franchises, management or marketing service contracts, non-equity cooperative arrangements and equity joint ventures. Inkpen also notes that by the late 1980s, ownership-based joint investments were considered to be a synonym for strategic alliances, but that from 1990s on, significance of other different forms of cooperation has started to grow.

A viewpoint similar to this is given by Grant and Baden-Fuller (2004: 62) who state that ''*...strategic alliances embrace a diversity of collaborative forms*" covering supplier-buyer partnerships, outsourcing agreements, technical collaboration, joint research projects, shared new product development, shared manufacturing arrangements, common distribution arrangements, cross selling arrangements and franchising.

Finally, all the criteria mentioned above, which make it possible to distinguish between the types of strategic alliances are not a definite end of the list, because the dynamics of modern business environment leads to constant creation of new types of alliances and the disappearance of the old ones.

KNOWLEDGE TRANSFER AND ORGANIZATIONAL LEARNING IN STRATEGIC ALLIANCES: A REVIEW

Strategic alliances are not a novelty in the business world. For example, the partnership between Ford and Mazda dates back to the year 1931, when Toyo Corg Kogui (Mazda's predecessor) asked Ford Motor Company to help them develop three-wheel vehicles in Japan (Pelliceli, 2003:2). However, the factors of modern world such as globalization, intensive technical and technological changes as well as regional integrations, influenced increase in the use of alliances as a business mechanism that is both reliable and flexible. Living in the world where knowledge is a dominant resource of business success, companies extensively started to use strategic alliances as a mechanism of knowledge generation, acquisition, implementation, and acceleration.

Contemporary theory makes a clear distinction between the concepts of organizational learning and organizational knowledge: organizational knowledge is the result of learning process, as well as the basis of further learning. Knowledge is ''information that corresponds to a particular context" (Burton et al, 2006: 92), while learning is the development of knowledge base (Shrivastava, 1981). For a long time, knowledge transfer was equated with technology transfer. From that perspective, organizational learning from an alliance partner was understood as the transfer of knowledge through the transfer of technology, and alliances were used as an effective mechanism for the transfer and successful implementation of technical and technological knowledge, regardless of the fact whether these are of material (new machinery, for example), or non-material nature (new procedures, for example). Later research developed in two directions: (1) differentiating between technical knowledge and organizational knowledge and (2) differentiating between technology transfer and knowledge transfer. Technical knowledge embedded in technology is only a part of organizational overall knowledge that can be a subject of transfer. Besides technology, every organization possesses other knowledge, embedded in its other elements. By the beginning of 2000, management literature started to recognize three most important knowledge repositories: people, tasks and tools (Argote, Ingram, 2000). People repository of knowledge is represented with the members of organization, their individual knowledge and the knowledge embedded in their social network. Tasks represent organizational goals, aims and purposes. Tools include all technical components, hardware and software. Finally, all these elements of organization require different approach to knowledge transfer. Logically, technology transfer differentiated from knowledge transfer. Apart from understanding knowledge transfer as ''*the changes in existing technology or managerial practice within an organization for which these changes represent a novelty*" (Lindholm, 1997), there are also other forms of knowledge an alliance can lead to, such as (1) creating new or significant transformation on the level of the existing knowledge and (2) the implementation of the existing knowledge in a new and unexploited way. Authors that have been analyzing knowledge transfer point to it as a complex process which includes three key elements: (1) characteristics of the subjects involved in knowledge transfer, (2) characteristics of knowledge being transferred and (3) characteristics of the mechanisms used for knowledge transfer. Since the beginning of 2000s management literature has been occupied with knowledge management rather than with knowledge transfer. Burton and Obel (2004: 10) state that knowledge management is an organization design issue to improve the efficiency and effectiveness of an organization and its people by sharing knowledge and information.

Further on, we will conceptualize our research on the basis of three mayor areas in management studies: strategy, organization and people.

Strategy – Related Issues of Organizational Learning and Knowledge Transfer in Strategic Alliances

Motivation and Intentions

Organizations decide to enter strategic alliance when they realize that they are not able to carry out a specific business venture on their own, for technological, market or other reasons. That is why a general strategic goal and the cornerstone of forming an alliance is to attract resources in order to create certain values for the partners in a way and to an extent which would not be attainable by their individual efforts (Inkpen, 2001: 404). Although the creation of strategic alliance does not necessarily imply equal distribution of benefits between both partners, each of the partners has to make some benefits through the alliance, which are considered to be relevant (Porter, Fuller, 1986).

In the literature on strategic alliances several theories were developed, which discuss the motives for creating strategic alliances. Each of these perspectives analyzes forming alliances in comparison with other strategic options of hierarchy and market ventures, emphasizing a specific business area: strategic market advantage, the availability of resources, economic efficacy. In their comment on the theories of creating strategic alliances, Grant and Baden-Fuller (2004: 63) state that strategic alliances are a complex phenomenon in which more than one reason for creation is involved, so that individual theories for creating strategic alliances have no potential to involve all the different types of alliances.

Pennings (1985) explanation of strategy offers a frame for understanding strategic orientation towards learning in strategic alliances. He defines strategy by recognizing its three crucial meanings: (1) explicit strategy – statement of intent that constrains and directs subsequent activities, (2) implicit strategy – an action of major impact that constraints or directs subsequent activities, and (3) rationalized strategy – rationalization or social construction that gives meaning to prior activities. Child (2003) argues that there are basically two ways to recognize strategic orientation towards learning within strategic alliance: (1) learning can be formally recognized as the goal of alliance creation and formulated in the mission statement, which is the more explicit and more straightforward way, and (2) learning can be recognized as important because partners showed a clear intention to learn and acquire knowledge from one another. Hamel (1991) defines this as *''an intention to learn''* suggesting that the achieved level of learning within an alliance depends highly on the reasons why company has entered alliance in the first place, and whether it sees learning as one of its aims to achieve through alliance creation.

Collaboration vs Competition

Child (2003:662) as well as Khanna et al. (1994) point that learning in strategic alliances can take either the form of competitive or collaborative learning. Competitive learning within strategic alliances is best illustrated by a situation in which one partner enters an alliance with a clear intention to learn as much as possible from the other partner, that way imposing its individual learning to mutual learning within an alliance.

The starting point of competitive perspective of organizational learning is that partners have to make their own organizational knowledge available to the other side, in order to provide any kind of learning from each other. However, at the beginning or in the process of cooperation one or both partners can come to conclusion that it is more lucrative to take as much as they can as fast as they can from the partnership, and then to abandon the project and continue doing business independently. Not rarely, partners within an alliance start behaving in an opportunistic way and follow the principle ‘ *'learn as much as you can and run away*!"

In this case, alliances lose their main role of the polygon for cooperation and mutual learning and become "*learning races"* (Khanna et al, 1994).

Naturally, the partners never talk about this openly, but the very manner in which they fbehave clearly shows that the aim of creating an alliance is to internalize the partner's skills and knowledge (Hamel, 1991: 86).

The analysis of organizational learning and knowledge transfer from the perspective of cooperation points to the fact that learning can be viewed as (1) mutual learning between the two equal partners and (2) learning between the partners who are not at the same level of knowledge so that the relation can be best described as the one between a tutor and a student. Mutual learning between two equal partners occurs in those situations in which each partner has something to learn from the alliance and when both of them see an alliance as a way to improve their ways of doing business in terms of learning and teaching. Another case is when partners are not completely equal, but one takes the role of a learner and the other the role of a teacher (Hamel, 1991). The analyses carried out in transitional economies so far mainly regarded the companies from these economies as learners, and foreign partners as tutors in this process (Lyles, 2002; Lyles, Salk, 1996; Woodside, Somogyi, 1994).

The issue of success or failure of strategic alliances is fully affirmed in this context. An alliance is considered to be successful when the goals for which it was created are accomplished. However, in the process of setting the goals of an alliance, the partners can take an opportunistic attitude, on the surface stating one goal as the desired and at the same time hiding the real goal which they attempt to reach secretly. When an alliance fails much before than it was initially planned, the question arises whether the failure is due to the fact that one of the partners reached their goal - learned what wanted, and therefore is not further interested to continue the partnership (Hamel, 1991, Khanna et al., 1994).

Control and Governance

Control within strategic alliance represents an important issue of its functioning in each of the developmental stages. Numerous research papers address the significance of control in terms of success of an alliance (Tannenbaum, 1968; Killing, 1983; Geringer, Hebert, 1989; Yan, Graz, 1994; Child, Yan, Lu, 1997). Geringer and Hebert (1989) identified three aspects of control within strategic alliance: (1) the aspects of mechanisms of control that partners apply, (2) the aspect of the level of control that one of the partners can have over the other and (3) the level of the activities that are subject to control within an alliance. The first of the questions mentioned above basically illustrates the process of designing the system of control within an organization and implies the following two parts: (1) the design of formal control system and (2) the design of informal, trust-based control system.

The mechanisms of formal control are predictable, regular and include explicit transfer of information, while the mechanisms of informal control are non-explicit by their very nature and embedded into the specific organizational context.

The reason why control proves to be an important factor for the survival of an alliance is the fact that alliances are a very suitable area for an opportunistic behavior of partners, which may lead to the disclosure and the loss of one of the partners' critical knowledge, the source of their competitive advantages and consequently, their being completely eliminated from the business arena in a relatively simple manner.

In most cases, the authors who work on this aspect of doing business within alliances point to the importance of being cautious and to gradual dynamics of revealing business information to the business partner. They also warn about the danger of potential opportunism in the partner's behavior.

These authors also recommend using the logics of economic theory of transactional costs, which implies that high transactional costs caused by potentially opportunistic behavior of the partner can be reduced by means of clearly defined conditions of doing business in the contract, as well as by means of ownership-based governance structures (Muthusamy, White, 2005: 417; Kogut, 1988).

Such results correspond to the results of Lyles and Salk (1996) from the research carried out in Hungary. The results of their research confirmed the importance of ownership for organizational learning and knowledge transfer within strategic alliances and showed that the highest level of knowledge transfer and learning is achieved in the partnership with 50%-50% ownership structure, a somewhat lower level in joint ventures in which the foreign partner has the major role, and the lowest level of knowledge transfer and learning in joint ventures in which the domestic partner maintains the majority.

Organization - Related Issues of Organizational Learning and Knowledge Transfer in Strategic Alliances

When referring to organization (design) issues within one-organization framework, it is widely accepted to apply the approach of drawing an organizational chart, that way representing connections and ties between formal organizational units within organization. When organizations create an alliance, this logic seems to be inapplicable, because there might not be organizational structure to tighten the relationships between partners. This relationship is usually (expected to be) defined by an alliance contract. Therefore, a corresponding formal organizational chart cannot be drawn for an alliance. That brings about a new challenge into analysis of the role of organization (design) in strategic alliances. Literature recognizes the importance of absorptive capacity of the firm to receive and accept knowledge, as well as to promote learning process. The concept of absorptive capacities was developed by Cohen and Levinthal (1989, 1990). They define absorptive capacity as a firm's general ability to value, assimilate, and commercialize new, external knowledge. Child (2001: 659), for instance, says that companies must have" *"the experience or capacity to acquire and absorb knowledge available from the alliance partner"*. Lyles (2001: 681) draws on the importance of an ability to absorb knowledge by defining organizational learning as "*embedded know-how resulting from absorptive capacity, receptivity of the firm to new knowledge, and the firms ability to develop knowledge utilization skills"*. Szulanski (1996) notes that knowledge transfer is less difficult if recipients are prepared to receive that knowledge. Cohen and Levinthal (1990) refer to the same issue in a similar way explaining that transferability of knowledge is related to recipients ''absorptive capacity". Cummings relates to this issue by defining knowledge embeddedness as an extent to which knowledge is held within organizational routines, systems and social networks (Cummings, 2001:212). Hamel (1991: 87) recognizes the importance of organizational ability to receive knowledge by defining receptivity as a determinant of learning. According to him, receptivity is a function of the skills and absorptiveness of receptors, exposure of position and parallelism in facilities, while asymmetry in receptivity pre-ordains asymmetric learning. Lane and Lubatkin (1998) relate the absorptive capacity to receptivity and suggest that absorptive capacity of a firm depends on the relevance of the student firm's basic knowledge to the teacher's firm knowledge base, the similarities in organizational structures of teaching and learning firms, and the similarity of the student and teacher firms' compensation practices.

Besides the research on absorptive capacity, and Child's thorough analysis (Child, 2003), the knowledge on the influence of inter-organizational design of an alliance on organizational learning and knowledge transfer is weak in particular. As Inkpen and Ramaswamy note

> "Even though many studies have argued that the ability to transfer knowledge is a primary source of a firm's competitive advantage and growth, we know relatively little about how to transfer knowledge within and across organizational boundaries" (2006: 108).

In the work of Nonaka, Tayoma and Byosiere (2001: 498) we find the unique explanation that seems to be quite helpful in explaining the logics of the idea of interorganizational design as a frame for partners' interactions and knowledge flows. The foundation of their theory of learning is in the Japanese philosophy, further applied to the concept of knowledge.

They introduce concept of *Ba,* and define it as a "*place where knowledge is shared, created and utilized*", "*a framework in which knowledge is activated as a resource*". Further, they explain that *Ba* does not necessarily mean space in physical terms, but covers virtual space (e-mail, teleconferences) and mental space (shared experience, ideas, etc.) as well, and the combination of those. In their view, Ba functions as *"a platform for the concentration of organization's knowledge assets"* with the potentials to capture the diffusion and dynamism of knowledge and learning process.

Organization science research also showed interest in the investigation of knowledge transfer efficiency of various organizational mechanisms, such as rotations of employees and managers, meetings, joint training and development programs, the use of modern communications based on the Internet and other telecommunication platforms, and the development of shared vision and organization culture.

The results of all this research signify that knowledge transfer success depends on the achieved level of fit between the type of knowledge to be transferred, mechanisms used for that purpose, and the characteristics of subjects involved in that transfer of knowledge. In her research Kostova (1999) showed the importance of respecting differences between different countries.

Overcoming the well known Hofstede's findings on the influence of national culture, she emphasized the influence of institutional differences and organizational practices which reflect these differences. Kostova concluded that even in the cases when certain practices are successfully transferred across national borders, there is a possibility that they will simply not fit into institutional environment and therefore the results will fail.

People- Related Issues of Organizational Learning and Knowledge Transfer in Strategic Alliances

Together with the characteristics of knowledge being transferred and the characteristics of mechanisms used for knowledge transfer (previously explained), authors that have been analyzing knowledge transfer in an alliance context particularly emphasize the importance of characteristics of subjects involved in knowledge transfer. The term "subjects" in this case should and can be understood in two ways – on organizational level (partners) and individual (people) level. Though often neglected in management research, people related issues proved to be of high importance for organizational learning and knowledge transfer in strategic alliances.

Dodgson's research (1993), for example, primarily focused on technological aspects of cooperation but the results turned researcher's attention to the importance and the role of trust in this process. According to these results, technological cooperation among companies is always followed by problems which are interpersonal in nature, and which can be overcome only through investing in building trust based on mutual interests, organizational cultures which are opened one to another, and informing employees about the status and aims of the partnership. Relationship quality is also recognized as important in the work of Ariño and de la Torre (1998). Inkpen and Ramaswamy (2006) note that trust is the key word for the success of an alliance. Numerous research point to different aspects of the influence that trust can have on strategic alliances (Yan, Gray, 1994; Ariño, de la Torre, 1998; Child, Faulkner, 1998; Inkpen, Currall, 1998; Inkpen, Ramaswamy, 2006).

Table I. Key research on organizational learning in strategic alliances

Source	Area	Research method	Results and conclusions
Pucik (1991)	*Technology Transfer in Strategic Alliances: Competitive Collaboration and Organizational Learning*	Theoretical	Problems with learning in strategic alliances and the absence of learning are the result of inadequate efforts of managers in planning and enabling conditions for learning.
Hamel (1991)	*Competition for Competence and Interpartner Learning within International Strategic Alliances*	Empirical	The level of learning that will be achieved through the alliance depends on the reasons for which alliance was created and whether learning is recognized as an alliance goal. Partners can have mutually competing goals. Different forms of knowledge have at the same time different transparency, so asymmetric learning results from asymmetric availability of different forms of knowledge.
Parkhe (1991)	*Interfirm Diversity, Organizational Learning and Longevity in Global Strategic Alliances*	Theoretical	Development of a multilevel typology of inter-firm diversity. Research is focused on organizational learning and adaptation as critical processes that dynamically moderate diversity's impact on alliance longevity and effectiveness.
Mody (1993)	*Learning Through Alliances*	Theoretical	Alliances are instable business ventures, so it is essential to keep them flexible. There is a trade off between flexibility and weak incentive structure of the alliance. Although the principle goal of the experimental set-up is to learn more about technical and market parameters, learning also occurs about working in an alliance and could lead to greater competence in managing alliances, partially alleviating incentive problems.
Dodgson (1993)	*Learning, Trust and Technological Cooperation*	Empirical	Technological cooperation of companies is inevitable followed by interpersonal problems. These problems can be overcome by building mutual trust based on joint interests, opened organizational cultures and informing employees about the static and the aims of the partnership.
Inkpen, Crossan (1995)	*Joint Ventures and Organizational Learning*	Empirical	Conceptual framework for studying organizational learning in joint ventures. Managerial learning, share and integration of managerial knowledge into organizational context, institutionalization of learning and influence of learning on performances are seen as the key issues.

Table I. (Continued)

Source	Area	Research method	Results and conclusions
Mowery, Oxley, and Silverman (1996)	*Strategic Alliances and Interfirm Knowledge Transfer*	Theoretical	Alliances based on ownership are more effective than contractual in those situations when it is necessary to transfer complex competences.
Powell, Koput, Smith-Doerr (1996)	*Inter-organizational Collaboration and the Locus of Innovation: Networks of Learning in Biotechnology*	Empirical	Investigation of organizational learning from the network perspective, which connects research on alliances in biotechnology with the following factors (1) experience in managing inter-organizational relationships, (2) network position, (3) growth rate and (4) portfolio of common activities.
Makhija and Ganesh (1997)	*The Relationship Between Control and Partner Learning in Learning Oriented Joint Ventures*	Theoretical	The model developed draws on resource-based, information-processing, and organizational learning theories to show how JV control processes affect the dynamics of interpartner learning. According to the model, firms forming learning-related JVs match with partners in line with their differences in capability and other requirements; the result is referred to as the asymmetry-need configuration. The model emphasizes that JVs with learning objectives are inherently and inevitably dynamic because of these internal processes.
Inkpen, Dinur (1998)	*Knowledge Management processes and International Joint Ventures*	Empirical	The authors examine the processes used by alliance partners to transfer knowledge from an alliance context to a partner context. They identify four key processes-technology sharing, alliance-parent interaction, personnel transfers, and strategic integration-that share a conceptual underpinning and represent a knowledge connection between parent and alliance. Although all of the knowledge management processes are potentially effective, the different processes involve different types of knowledge and different organizational levels. The results suggest that although a variety of knowledge management strategies can be viable, some strategies lead to more effective knowledge transfer than others.

Source	Area	Research method	Results and conclusions
Inkpen, (1998)	*Learning, Knowledge Acquisition and Strategic Alliances*	Theoretical	Learning through strategic alliances is demanding, frustrating and often misunderstood process. Creation of good learning environment in strategic alliances is an exception more than a rule.
Lane, Lubatkin (1998)	*Relative Absorptive Capacity and Inter-organizational Learning*	Empirical	One firm's ability to learn from another firm is argued to depend on the similarity of both firms' (1) knowledge bases, (2) organizational structures and compensation policies, and (3) dominant logics.
Kumar and Nti (1998)	*Differential Learning and Interaction in Alliance Dynamics*	Theoretical	This research develops a dynamic theory of alliances by examining certain outcome and process discrepancies that may emerge as the partners interact. Outcome and process discrepancies may emerge as collaboration unfolds. How the partners assess and react to discrepancies shapes the developmental path of an alliance. Guidelines for assessing and managing outcome and process discrepancies are suggested.
Larsson, Bengtsson, Henriksson and Spark (1998)	*The Inter-organizational Learning Dilemma: Collective Knowledge Development in Strategic Alliances*	Theoretical	This research focuses on the dilemma of opportunistic individual learning and collective learning under conditions of inter-organizational cooperation. The way partners manage the collective learning process plays the central role in the success and failure of strategic alliances. Five different learning strategies are developed.
Arinjo, de la Tore (1998)	*Learning from Failure: Towards an Evolutionary Model of Collaborative Ventures*	Empirical	Authors develop a model of collaborative processes in alliances. They conclude that positive feedback loops are critical in the evolutionary process, that relationship quality is both an outcome and a mediating variable, and that procedural issues are critical from the start in fostering a climate for positive reinforcement and the building of mutual trust and confidence in the relationship.
Simonin (1997, 1999)	*Collaboration and Learning Organizations*	Empirical	Experience alone is insufficient for the achievement of the greatest benefits from collaboration. Experience must be internalized first, and collaborative know-how must be developed for this experience to contribute to future collaborative benefits.
Lyles (2001)	*Organizational learning in international joint ventures*	Empirical	The analysis of student-teacher relationship in strategic alliances functioning within transition economies. The role of foreign partners is critical in enabling training, technology, financial resources and marketing skills.

Table I. (Continued)

Source	Area	Research method	Results and conclusions
Iyer (2002)	*Learning in Strategic Alliances: An Evolutionary Perspective*	Theoretical	Development of evolutionary model of learning in strategic alliances.
Child, (2003)	*Learning through strategic alliances*	Theoretical	Partners need to show intention to learn through an alliance. Partners need to have adequate learning capacities for accepting new knowledge and abilities to manage the process of knowledge acquisition.
Ghosh, (2004)	*Learning in strategic alliances-a Vygotskian perspective*	Theoretical	Socio-cultural-historical perspective on strategic alliances which offers an improvement of theoretical framework of learning in alliances.
Grant, Baden-Fuller (2004)	*A knowledge accessing theory of strategic alliances*	Theoretical	Authors argue that the primary advantage of alliances over both firms and markets is in *accessing* rather than *acquiring* knowledge. Building upon the distinction between the knowledge generation ('exploration') and knowledge application ('exploitation'), they show that alliances contribute to the efficiency in the application of knowledge; first, by improving the efficiency with which knowledge is integrated into the production of complex goods and services, and second, by increasing the efficiency with which knowledge is utilized.
Muthusamy, White, (2005)	*Learning and Knowledge Transfer in Strategic Alliances: A Social Exchange View*	Empirical	Drawing on social exchange theory, we examined the effects of social exchange processes between alliance partners on the extent of learning and knowledge transfer in a strategic alliance. An empirical examination shows that social exchanges such as reciprocal commitment, trust, and mutual influence between partners are positively related to learning and knowledge transfer in strategic alliances..
Becerra, Lunnan and Huemer (2008)	*Trustworthiness, Risk and the transfer of tacit and explicit knowledge between alliance partners.*	Empirical	Explicit knowledge is closely associated with the firm's willingness to take risk, tacit knowledge is intimately related to high trustworthiness. The results support the important role of trust and the transfer of tacit knowledge on the success of learning alliances.
Meier, (2011)	*Knowledge Management in Strategic Allainces: A RFeview of Empirical Evidence*	Theoretical - Review paper	The paper offers a review of empirical evidence on knowledge management in strategic alliances.

The main idea of this type of research is to question the influence that trust between partners has on the level of organizational learning and knowledge transfer. Theoretically, it is expected that the increase in the level of trust between partners will simultaneously result with the increase in their willingness to make their knowledge available and to share their knowledge; at the same time, it is expected that the probability that one of the partners will behave in an opportunistic manner and make use of the other will decrease.

Trust is, in that manner highly associated with the "relationship risks", as defined by Paik[2]. The term "relationship risks" implies the danger that the other side will not strictly stick to the initially set conditions and obligations. However, there are only few in the present corpus that directly focus on the relation between trust and organizational learning within alliances.

Among these that exclusively focus on the role of trust for learning in strategic alliances, two specifically stand out, as they came to completely opposite results. The first is the research into trust and inter-organizational learning in the inter-organizational joint ventures in Hungary.

The research was done by Lane and associates (1998) and did not report statistically relevant dependence between trust and learning, but did report statistically relevant dependence between trust and performance.

Nevertheless, a recent research published by Muthusamy and White (2005) approaches the concept of trust from the perspective of social exchange. Their research reported that trust between partners has a strong influence on the process of learning between the partners. Mutual devotion depends on moral responsibility of a partner, and heavily reflects learning in strategic alliances.

Previous experience is also recognized as a supportive factor inalliance learning processes. Child (2003: 669) explains that previous experience with managing alliances, as well as having collaborated with the same partner before positively influences learning through alliances. Our recent study (Aleksić Mirić, 2011) also confirms the importance of previous experience in managing knowledge in alliances.

Knowledge Transfer and Organizational Learning in Strategic Alliances: Research Perspectives

On the basis of performed theoretical research, we can notice that in the area of managing strategic alliances certain research gaps and inconsistencies can be recognized. However, the existing knowledge demonstrates the need for improvement both in conceptual and empirical research. On the line of the identified key research areas, we suggest further research in: strategic orientation towards learning and strategic fit, organizational structure and design, organizational network analysis, influence of incentives system and organizational culture and climate.

---

[2] Paik (2005: 490) defines two main types of risks involved in any kind of alliances: (1) relationship risks and (2) performance risks. Relationship risk is highly characteristic of strategic alliances, because in case of mergers and acquisitions relationship risk is completely reduced. Performance risk is characteristic of all kinds of strategic decisions, due to the fact that in each business venture there is some uncertainty about its outcome.

Strategy – Related Issues

Strategic Orientation towards Learning and Strategic Fit

Some companies recognize the importance of learning and emphasize it in a way so as to clearly and unambiguously include it in strategy statement. Others use a less transparent manner and do not include learning in the formulation of strategy- it is the underlying pattern of strategic decisions made regarding the functioning of an alliance that undoubtedly reflects strategic orientation towards learning. Finally, the deepest level of acceptance of learning as a strategic objective is in the third case, when people in alliance recognize learning as their own, inner value. In alliances, the positions of organizational knowledge and organizational learning are often very different. When alliances are created, very often the existing organizational knowledge of each of the partners is the subject of financial evaluation. Especially in case of equity-based alliances, partners express the individual knowledge-capital they bring into the deal. In transition countries, for instance, in equity-based alliances formation, organizational knowledge is often recognized as the most valuable investment by partners. However, the contract between the partners very often fail to define precisely what that investment involves, or if there is an action plan to specify what knowledge transfer covers.

Implication 1a: The awareness of and the intention to learn from the partnership are the pre-conditions of organizational learning. Without them, any learning resulting from an alliance is an uncontrolled coincidence.

Research gap 1a: Research on learning in strategic alliances should be more precise about strategic intentions towards learning and the position of learning within alliance goals, especially in case of non research and development alliances.

The second important theme in strategy research regarding strategic alliances refers to strategic complementarities between partners: does the combination of the skills and resources allow the alliance entity to perform a task that could not be performed that well by the partners acting alone – i.e. strategic fit (Inkpen, Ramaswamy, 2006). The concept of fit is well recognized and used in organizational theory. Different authors have been using this concept in order to test the relationship between two (or more) organizational variables. On the one hand, a large body of literature is dedicated to this subject, resulting in a remarkable body of knowledge; on the other hand, that knowledge is unconnected, and separately analyzes the relationships between few variables, with no intentions to offer integrative model. Burton et al., (2002) demonstrated that those organizations that fit better perform better. The concept of fit has been mostly analyzed from one-organization perspective, i.e. how to achieve those integrative elements of organization (contingency factors and elements of organization design) align one to another. In the area of strategic alliances, the concept of fit has not been implemented as much as it seems it has potentials to explain various phenomena regarding alliance functioning.

Strategic fit refers to strategic complementarities between partners: does the combination of skills and resources allow an alliance entity to perform a task that could not be performed that well by partners acting alone? (Inkpen, Ramaswamy, 2006: 95). Strategic fit also deals with the question whether partners see the aim and the intentions of the partnership in the same way, and if they recognize the same objectives as the goals of partnership creation. Literature review shows that there is a high level of correlation between the potential level of learning within the partnership, and the choice of a partner. In other words, the higher the level of strategic compatibility between the partners, the higher the probability of significant knowledge transfer and organizational learning. On the other hand, there are works which are rather skeptical about the significance that strategic compatibility and careful selection of the partner have for the success of partnership. In support to these views it is augmented that a large number of alliances were formed between the partners quite different in their characteristics. In addition to this, theoretical analysis does not clearly show whether organizational potential of a company to learn and its potential to teach and transfer knowledge result from the good choice of the partner, or from carefully planned and carried out adaptation.

The results of this research confirm the significance of the selection process of the partner and its influence on further functioning and the success of a partnership. If a non-compatible organization is chosen in the process of selection, it is unlikely that organizational adaptation can make up for it. The process of organizational adaptation is very demanding and operationally complicated, so if it is loaded with wrong decisions made in the previous stage (that of selection) the likelihood of strategic partnership success decreases significantly. The most important element in the process of organizational learning and knowledge transfer is the partners' attitude to formulating the strategy of partnership and the strategic compatibility between the partners. The previous theoretical results provide some guidelines regarding strategic orientation towards learning.

Implication 1b: Strategic alignment (fit) between partners about organizational learning as one of the goals of partnership creation is the prerequisite for effectiveness of the mechanisms used for organizational learning and knowledge transfer.

Research gap 1b: Research on learning in strategic alliances should address the measurement of strategic fit between allies.

Organization – Related Issues

Organizational Structure and Design Fit

Inkpen and Ramaswamy (2006: 95) define organizational fit in terms of factors that stand for it and promote it, such as: common or similar corporate cultures and values, convergence of strategic goals, good chemistry between key managers, partners that value public reputation, compatible control and decision making systems, common time horizons, partners that discourage secretive behavior in their own operations. Broadly, organizational fit refers to the ability of partners to work together. Lorange and Rose (1991) recognize the importance of mutual adjustment of partnering organizations in strategic and organizational sense by identifying three fundamental reasons why strategic alliances are so difficult to manage. According to them (1) shared decision making, (2) separate corporate cultures and (3) different (conflicting) strategic interests are the main reasons for difficulties in managing strategic alliances. Although previous explanations are relevant and wide-covering, it seems that there is a lack of straightforward and unambiguous criteria that would define what elements compose an organization so that, on those basis, we could include some elements of organization as ''acceptable properties" (Burton, Obel, 2004: 24), and exclude others.

Theoretical research does not reveal if organization design contributes to organizational learning in strategic alliances, nor what the reasons that make organization design an important element in the process of knowledge transfer and learning in the alliance context are. Organizational design is dominantly studied as an inter-organizational issue, without recognizing its explicit potential to influence organizational learning and knowledge transfer in strategic alliances. The authors who did recognize the potential influence of the internal factors (among these, organizational structure as well) on the processes within alliances mainly use a very wide term *the absorptive capacity* of a company to gain and provide knowledge. A paper of Lane and Lubatkin (1998) offers more significant results on the influence of organizational structure and learning. In the research, the authors investigated the hypothesis that the similarity in organizational structures between the learning and the teaching partner is positively connected to inter-organizational learning, and did not find strong support for this argumentation. However, the way organizational structure is operationalized in the paper of Lane and Lubatkin leaves space for further inspections of the role and influence of organizational structure in alliance learning processes, especially in the domain of the influence that structural similarity has on organizational learning and knowledge transfer in alliances. It seems that the application of traditional understanding of organizational design is not potent enough to help us find answers to all these questions.

Together with traditional measures of organizational design, non-traditional measures based on organizational network analysis should be used in order to help us uncover the role of organizational design in learning processes in strategic alliances. Inter-organizational level of analysis (alliance settings) calls for regarding organizations as systems of communication channels and information processing system, composed of certain number of unites and structured in a way to fulfill predefined goal (consistently with RG1 and Implication 1). Research on organizational learning in strategic allainces can benefit more from the involvent of social network analysis. Network analysis gives additional inputs for considering the role of organization design in alliance knowledge transfer and learning: it enabled scheme representation of relationships and connections within networks in a way that could not be achieved with the standard organizational chart. It also allows for a deeper understanding of the role that organization design has in learning through strategic alliances, and gives the possibility to measure relationships between subjects, that cannot be seen on standard organization scheme and measured in a different way. Network analysis gives an opportunity to view organizations from the perspective of connections among organizations' members. Analysis alike has two basic functions: (1) it represents the relationship between partners by quantifying and presenting scheme information flow channels, that are in fact carriers of learning, and (2) it gives us the possibility to construct a flow-chart, which is an advanced form of the traditional organizational scheme applied on inter-organizational level. This analysis also enables to represent and observe what Nonaka et al. marked as *Ba* and define as "*a place where knowledge is shared, created and utilized*"

Implication 2: Strategic and organization design fit between allies define organizational capacities and capabilities to acquire and absorb knowledge – i.e. define alliance's absorptive capacity for learning.

Organization design puts frames within which knowledge circulates moves and modifies. When referring to multi-organizational perspective, as in the case of alliances, organization design defines both organizations' ability to accept and to give knowledge. Since both giving and getting knowledge ask for some mechanisms by which knowledge is transferred, organization design defines the paths and routes of this transfer as well.

Research gap 2a: Research on learning in strategic alliances should be more precise about the role of organizational design and influence its properties have on learning and knowledge transfer in the alliance context.

Research gap 2b: Research on learning in strategic alliances should address the measurement of organizational fit between allies.

The Influence of Organizational Compensations

In economics theory, incentive is defined as "any factor (financial or non-financial) that provides a motive for a particular course of action, or counts as a reason for preferring one choice to the alternatives". Incentives can be designed in a way to support individual or group action towards a certain goal. The idea that the design of incentive system has important implications on the fulfillment of alliance goals has not been widely recognized among practitioners, nor among theoreticians. There are a number of reasons and potential answers to the question why rewarding system is neglected when managing alliances. Yashino and Rangan (1995:163) explain that "*...incentive systems deeply embedded in the fabric of organizations are built over years in response to past needs; alliances are too recent, and too unique to be easily incorporated into traditional incentive system.*" Besides recognizing incentives as an important part of managing alliances, incentives have not been widely recognized as a *"vital component to design of the firm*" (Burton et al., 2006:182) as well. In most cases, authors have been connecting incentives to personnel management and accounting and rarely to organizational design activities. Recent trends in the area of organizational design support the idea that *"design of incentives goes hand-in-hand with all the other components of organizational design"* (Burton et.al., 2006:182). In economics theory, incentive is defined as "*any factor (financial or non-financial) that provides a motive for a particular course of action, or counts as a reason for preferring one choice to the alternatives*". Incentives can be designed in a way to support individual or group action towards a certain goal.

In the context of managing strategic alliances, incentives become an important part of stimulating and motivating people to: (1) accept alliance as a new form of organizational functioning and (2) recognize the goal of alliance creation and adjust behavior in a way to support fulfillment of that goal. The basic logic for this is that by rewarding certain forms of behavior management can enhance and motivate people to behave in such a way. The most important thing for management therefore is to recognize the forms of behavior that support presupposed management goals and to reward these types of behavior by designing appropriate incentive scheme. At the moment, the influence of incentive system on organizational learning and knowledge transfer in strategic alliances is not investigated enough. Lane and Lubatkin (1998) did find support for the argument that similarity in partners' incentive systems (in case of a teacher-learner relationship) is positively associated with interorganizational learning. Incentive system is especially ignored as a mechanism for achieving certain alliance goals, and most of all, the goal of learning. Strategic alliances seem to be a fertile ground for "*rewarding A while hoping for B*" mistake (Kerr, 1986) to occur.

Implication 3: The influence of incentive system on organizational learning and knowledge transfer in strategic alliances is under investigation. Incentive system is very important, but ignored especially as a mechanism for achieving certain alliance goals, and most of all, for the goal of learning.

Research gap 3: Research on learning in strategic alliances should address the influence that non-financial and financial incentive systems have on learning and transfer of knowledge.

People – Related Issues

Lorange and Rose (1991) recognize the importance of good climate towards strategic alliance within an organization as one of the things that might significantly influence the success of partnership, saying that "*...during the more intense formation phases [management should ensure] that a broad range of people within the organization is committed to and enthusiastic about the venture*". Recent research carried out by Wijk, Jansen and Lyles (2007) reports that when organizations share unique systems of values, higher knowledge transfer can be achieved, while organizations that are culturally distant can have lower potential for knowledge transfer. Theoretical knowledge, research and practice all confirm that good climate towards the partnership creation, and fit in cultural dimensions are important for partnership success in various stages. Findings also support the idea that behavioral aspects of strategic partnership can be put aside during its planning phase, but they will certainly arise during implementation (Walter, 1985; Berry, 1993; Nahavandi, Malekzadeh, 1986, 1988, 1990; Anderson, 1995). This phenomenon was identified as ''*collision of cultures*": differences in philosophy behind doing business because of different basic assumptions about the mission, strategy and aims of organization, which manifest as differences in systems of values and attitudes of managers and employees and consequently cause differences in behavior.

Implication 4: Cultural misfits per se do not imply that cultures will necessarily collide, causing organizational misfit that will negatively affect organizations' potentials to learn one from another. The likelihood that cultural misfit will result in a collision of cultures might be mediated by other factors, among which type of industry is the most important.

Research gap 4: Research on learning in strategic alliances should investigate both positive and negative effects of differences in cultures that cause organizational misfits among allies, in the light of their influence on learning and knowledge transfer.

CONCLUSION

As the beginning of XXI century has indicated, the empirical data available today confirm that further development of the world market moves in the direction of linking companies and their cooperation at different levels. While companies are completely aware of the need to cooperate and work jointly, at the same time they fight to keep relatively independent position and to achieve strategically important goals through loosely-coupling with others. In that atmosphere, strategic alliances as the form of inter-firm cooperation start gaining importance. Another parallel trend that has embraced the world market is the domination of knowledge as the basic resource of competitive advantage. The business world today is built on the assumption that one can be better than one's competition if knows. In that global race for competiveness, companies often decide to enrich their knowledge and strengthen their competitive advantages by forming strategic alliances. Nevertheless, business venture might not succeed to justify targeted goals, and may even jeopardize company's well being.

Organizational learning and knowledge transfer in strategic alliances happen in the process of interaction among partners. Even in cases when alliances are not created with specific learning motivation, learning processes spontaneously happen as partners interact. However, the outcomes of such systematically unmanaged learning are not necessarily positive. This chapter was systematized in a way to explain that knowledge management processes in strategic alliances should be carefully managed on strategic, organizational, and people level. The existing knowledge confirms that the awareness of and the intention to learn from the partnership are the pre-conditions of organizational learning. Strategic alignment between partners about organizational learning as one of the goals of partnership creation is seen as a prerequisite for effectiveness of the mechanisms used for organizational learning and knowledge transfer. However, empirical research did incline towards focusing on research and development alliances, as the most explicit case of learning alliances, while others are less investigated.

The existing research predominantly focused on the alliance absorptive capacity. As we see it, strategic and organization design fit between allies define organizational capacities and capabilities to acquire and absorb knowledge – i.e. define alliance's absorptive capacity for learning. The existing knowledge is particularly modest in the domain of influence organizational design has for knowledge management processes in strategic alliances. Further research should be more precise about the role of organizational design, and influence its properties have on learning and knowledge transfer in the alliance context. It should be more explicit in two directions: the investigation of the influence of incentive system, and the analysis of organizational networks. Existing knowledge implies to an extent that successful learning in alliances depends on people motivation. Still, a significant gap is recognized in the domain of the influence of incentive system on organizational learning and knowledge transfer in strategic alliances. Incentive system is very important, but ignored especially as a mechanism for achieving certain alliance goals, and most of all, for the goal of learning, an further research should address this issue with more care.

Organization design puts frames within which knowledge circulates moves and modifies. When referring to multi-organizational perspective, as in the case of alliances, organization design defines both organizations' ability to accept and to give knowledge. Since both giving and getting knowledge ask for some mechanisms by which knowledge is transferred, organization design defines the paths and routes of this transfer as well. It is possible that the lack of research on the design influence comes as the consequence of understanding organizational design as an exclusively inter-organizational issue. A standard way of organizational analysis relying on traditional organizational dimensions does not have adequate analytical potentials when dealing with inter-organizational processes, but organizations need to be approached from another perspective, network perspective. Partnerships might not have their organizational chart, but they have flowcharts which managers should be aware of. Network analysis enables the analysis of relationship structure between partners, while the use of statistical and computational models enables quantitative expressions of images within these relationships and connections. Further research should benefit from the application of network perspective on learning in strategic alliances, measurement and interpretation it offers. Successful knowledge management in strategic alliances does not depend on the similarity of partners, but on their ability to achieve strategic, organizational and cultural fit.

REFERENCES

Aleksić Mirić, A., „Influence of Network Maturity on Organizational Learning and Knowledge Transfer in Strategic Alliances" (pg 317-337) in *New Developments in the Theory of Networks: Franchising, Alliances and Cooperatives*, Tuunanen, M.; Windsperger, J.; Cliquet, G.; Hendrikse, G. (Eds.), 1st Edition., 2011, XI, 390 p.

Ariño, A., de la Torre, J., Ring, P.S., (2001), »Relational Quality: Managing Trust in Corporate Alliances«, *California Management Review*, Vol.44, No1: 109-121

Ariño, A., Reuer, J.J., (2004), ''Designing And Renegotiating Strategic Alliance Contract", *Academy of Management Executive*, Vol.18, No.3.

Burton, M.R., DeSanctis, G., Obel, B., (2006), Organisational *Design: A Step by Step Approach*, Cambridge.

Burton, M.R., Obel, B., (2004), *Strategic* Organisational *Diagnosis and Design: The Dynamics of Fit*, Springer.

Burgers, W.P., Hill, C.W., Chan Kim, W., (1993), »A Theory of Global Strategic Alliance: the Cae of the Global Auto Industry«, *Strategic Management Journal*, Vol.14, 419-432.

Child, J. , Markoczy, L. (1993). Host-country managerial behaviour and learning in Chinese and Hungarian joint ventures. *Journal of Management Studies*, 30, pp. 611–631.

Child, J., Czeglédy, A., (1996), »Managerial Learning in the Transformation of Eastern Europe: Some Key Issues«, *Organization Studies*, 17/2, 167-179.

Child, J., Rodrigues, S., (1996) The Role of Social Identity in the International Transfer of Knowledge through Joint Ventures in S.R. Clegg and G.Palmer (eds), Producing Management Knowledge, London, Sage, 46-68.

Child, J., Yan, Y., Lu, Y., (1997), »Ownership and Control in Sino-Foreign Joint Ventures« u Beamish, P., Killing, J., (eds) *Cooperative Strategies: Asian Pacific Perspective*, San Francisco, California: New Lexington, 181-225.

Child, J., (2003), ''Learning Through Strategic Alliances", in *Handbook of* Organisational learning *and Knowledge*, Oxford University Press: 657-680.

Cummings, J., (2001), Knowledge Transfer Across RandD Units: An Empirical Investigation Of The Factors Affecting Successful Knowledge Transfer Across Intra And Inter Organisational Units, doctoral dissertation, George Washington University, Washington DC.

Cohen, W. M., Levinthal, D. A., (1989), ''Innovation and Learning: The Two Faces of RandD", *Economic Journal*, 99: 569-590.

Dierkes, M., Bethoin A.A., Child, J., Nonaka, I., (2001), *Handbook of* Organisational learning, Oxford University Press.

Doz, Y.L., (1996), "The Evolution of Cooperation in Strategic Alliances: Initial Conditions or Learning Processes?", *Strategic Management Journal*, Vol.17, 55-83.

Dodgson, M., (1993), ''Learning, Trust and Technological Cooperation", *Human Relations*, 46:77-95.

Fiol,C.M., Lyles, M.A., (1985), ''Organisational learning", *Academy of Management Review*, 10 (4): 803-813.

Geringer, J.M., Hebert, L., Control and Performance of International Joint Ventures, *Journal of International Business Studies,* Vol. 20, No. 2 (Summer, 1989), pp. 235-254.

Grant, R.M., Baden-Fuller,C., (2004), ''A Knowledge Accessing Theory of Strategic Alliances", *Journal of Management Studies*, January, 41:1.

Grant, R.M., (1996), "Toward a knowledge based theory of the firm", *Strategic Management Journal*, Vol.17, 109-122.

Gulati, R., (1998), »Alliances and Networks«, *Strategic Management Journal*, Vo. 19, 293-317.

Hagendoorn, J., (1993), "Understanding the Rationale of Strategic Technology Partnering: International Modes of Cooperation and Sectoral Differences", *Strategic Management Journal*, 38: 85-112.

Hall, P.D., Norburn D, (1987), ''The Management Factor in Acquisition Performance", *Leadership and* Organisational *Development Journal*, 8.

Hamel,G., (1991), ''Competition for Competence and Interpartenr Learning within International Strategic Alliances", *Strategic Management Journal*, Vol.12, pp. 83-103.

Hamel, G., Doz, Y. L., Prahalad, C. K., (1989), ''Collaborate with your competitors--and win", *Harvard Business Review*, 67(1): 133-139.

Hamel, G., Prahald, C., (1994) *Competing for the Future*, Boston: Harvard Business School Press.

Hedberg, B., (1981), "How Organizations Learn and Unlearn", in Starbuck, W. (Ed.), *Handbook of* Organisational *Design*: 3-27. New York: Oxford University Press.

Hennart, J.F., (1988), "A Transaction Cost Theory of Equity Joint Ventures", *Strategic Management Journal*, 9: 361-374.

Hennart, J.F., Reddy, S. (1997),"The Choice Between Mergers, Acquisitions and Joint Ventures: The Case of Japanese Investors in the United States", *Strategic Management Journal*, 18: 1-12.

Huber. G.P., (1991), ''Organisational learning: the Contributing Process and the Literatures", *Organization Science*, Vol.2, No.1, February, 1991.

Inkpen, A.C. , Crossan, M.M. (1995). Believing is seeing: joint ventures and organizational learning. *Journal of Management Studies*, 32, pp. 595–618.

Inkpen, A.C., (1996), ''Creating Knowledge Through Collaboration", *California Management Review*, 39 (1): 123-140.

Inkpen, A. C., Beamish, P. W., (1997), ''Knowledge, Bargaining Power, and the Instability of International Joint Ventures", *Academy of Management Review*, 22: 177-202.

Inkpen, A., Currall, S.C., (1998), ''The Nature, Antecedents and Consequences of Joint Venture Trust", *Journal of International Management*, 4 1-20.

Inkpen, A.C., (1998), ''Learning and Knowledge Acquisition through International Strategic Alliances", *Academy of Management Executive*, 12 (4):69-80.

Inkpen, A.C., (1998), ''Learning, Knowledge Acquisition and Strategic Alliances", *European Management Journal*, Volume 16,No 2, pp. 223-229(7).

Inkpen, A.C., Dinur, A., (1998), ''Knowledge Management processes and International Joint Ventures", *Organization Science*, 9 (4): 454-468.

Inkpen, A.C., (2001), Strategic Allinaces (Chapter 15) in *Oxford Handbook of International Business* (eds. Rugman, A.M., Brewer, T.L.), Oxford Scholarship Online Monographies.

Inkpen, A.C., Tsang, E.W.K., (2005), ''Social Capital, Networks, and Knowledge Transfer", *Academy of Management Review*, Vol. 30, No. 1, 146-165.

Inkpen A, Ramaswamy K (2006) Global Strategy: Creating and Sustaining Advantage Across Borders. Oxford University Press.

Iyer, K.N.S., (2002), ''Learning in Strategic Alliances: An Evolutionary Perspective", *Academy of Marketing Science Review*, No.10.

Khanna, T., Gulati, R., Nohria, N.,(1994), ''Alliances as Learning Races", *Academy of Management Proceedings.*

Khanna, T., Gulati, R., Nohria, N., (1998), ''The Dynamics of Learning Alliances: Competition, Cooperation and Relative Scope", *Strategic Management Journal*, Vol. 19, 193-210.

Killing, J.P., (1983), *Strategies for Joint Venture Success,* New York: Praeger.

Kogut, B., (1988), ''Joint Ventures: Theoretical and Empirical Perspectives", *Strategic Management Journal*, 9: 319-322.

Kogut, B., (2000), "The Network as Knowledge: Generative Rules and the Emergence Structure", *Strategic Management Journal*, 21: 405-425.

Kostova, T., Transnational Transfer of Strategic Organizational Practices: A Contextual Perspective, *The Academy of Management Review*, Vol. 24, No. 2. (Apr., 1999), pp. 308-324.

Kumar, R., Nti, K.O., (1998), ''Differential Learning and Interaction in Alliance Dynamics", *Organization Science*, 37 (1): 19-33.

Lane, P., Lubatkin, M., (1998), ''Relative Absorptive Capacity and Inter-organisational learning", *Strategic Management Journal*, Vol. 19, pp. 461-477.

Lane, P., Salk, J., Lyles, M. A., (2001), ''Knowledge Acquisition and Performance In Transitional Economy International Joint Ventures", *Strategic Management Journal*, 22: 1139-1162.

Larsson, R., Bengtsson, L., Henriksson, K., Sparks, J., (1998), ''The Interorganisational learning Dilemma: Collective Knowledge Development in Strategic Alliances", *Organization Science*, 9: 285-305.

Levinthal, D.A., March, J.G., (1993), ''The Myopia of Learning", *Strategic Management Journal*, Vol. 14, 95-112.

Lindholm, N., (1997), ''Learning Processes in International Joint Ventures in China", *Advances in Chinese Industrial Studies*, 5: 193-54.

Lorange, P., Roos, J., (1991), "Why Some Strategic Alliances Succeed and Others Fail", *Journal of Business Strategy*, January-February, 25-30.

Luo, Y., 1997, ''Partner Selection and Venturing Success: The Case of Joint Ventures With Firms in The People's Republic of China", *Organization Science*, 8: 648-662.

Lyles, M. A., (1988), "Learning Among Joint Venture Sophisticated Firms", Management International Review, 28(Special Issue): 85-97.

Lyles, M. A., Salk, J. E., (1996), "Knowledge Acquisition from Foreign Parents in International Joint Ventures: An Empirical Examination in the Hungarian Context", *Journal of International Business Studies*, 27: 877-904.

Lyles, M., (2003), ''Organisational learning in International Joint Ventures: The Case of Hungary", in *Handbook of* Organisational learning *and Knowledge*, Oxford University Press: 657-680.

Makhija, M.V., Ganesh, U., (1997), ''The Relationship Between Control and Partner Learning in Learning Oriented Joint Ventures", *Organization Science*, 5: 508-520.

Mowery, D.C., Oxley, J.E., Silverman, B.S., (1996), Strategic Alliances and Interfirm Knowledge Transfer, *Strategic Management Journal*, Vol.17 (winter special issue), pp:77-91.

Meier, M., (2011), Knowledge Management in Strategic Alliances: A Review of Empirical Evidence, International Journal of Management Reviews, Vol 13, 1-23.

Muthusamy SK, White MA (2006) Learning and knowledge transfer in strategic alliances: a social exchange view. Organ Stud 26(3):415–441

Nonaka, I., (1991), ''The Knowledge Creating Company", *Harvard Business Review*, Nov-Dec: 96.

Nonaka, I., (1994), ''A Dynamic Theory of Organisational Knowledge Creation", *Organization Science*, Vol, 5, No.1, 14-37.

Nonaka, I., Takeutchi, H., (1995), *The Knowledge Creating Company*, New York: McGrawHill.

Nonaka, i., Toyama, R., Byosiere, P., (2003), A Theory of Organizational Knowledge Creation: Understanding the Dynamic Process of Creating Knowledge in in *Handbook of* Organisational learning *and Knowledge*, Oxford University Press: 491-518

Osborn, R., Hagedoorn, J., (1997), "The Institutionalization and Evolutionary Dynamics of Interorganisational Alliances and Networks", *Academy of Management Journal*, Vol.40, No2, 261-278.

Parkhe, A, (1991), ''Interfirm Diversity, Organisational learning, and Longevity in Global Strategic Alliances", *Journal of International Business Studies*, 22: 579-601.

Pelliceli, A., (2003), »Strategic Alliances«, EADI Workshop "Clusters and global value chains in the north and the third world", Facoltà di Economia – Novara – 30/31 Ottobre 2003.

Polanyi, M., (1962), *Personal Knoweldge: Towards a post critical philo*sophy, New York: Harper Torchbooks.

Polanyi, M., (1966), *The Tacit Dimension*, London: Routledge and Kegan Paul.

Porter, M., Fuller, M.B., (1986), *Coalitions and Global Strategies* u Porter, M., (ed) *Competition In Global Industries,* Boston, Mass: Harvard Business School Press.

Pucik, V., (1991) ''Technology Transfer in Strategic Alliances: Competitive Collaboration and Organisational learning" in Agmon, T., VonGlinow, M.A., (eds) *Technology Transfer and International Business*, New York: Oxford University Press, 121-138.

Szulanski, G. (1996), Exploring Internal Stickiness: Impediments to the Transfer of Best Practice Within the Firm, Strategic Management Journal, Vol. 17, (Winter Special Issue), pp. 27-43.

Tannenbaum, A, (1968), Control in Organizations, New York> McGraw Hill.

Van Wijk, R., Jansen, J, Lyles, M., (2008), Inter- and Intra-Organizational Knowledge Transfer: A Meta-Analytic Review and Assessment of its Antecedents and Consequences, Journal of Management Studies, Vol45(4).

Woodside, AG, Somogyi, P. (1994), "Creating international joint ventures: strategic insights from case research on a successful Hungarian-Japanese industrial enterprise", in

Buckley, PJ, Ghauri, PN (Eds),The Economics of Change in East and Central Europe, Academic Press .

Yashino, M., Rangan, U.S., (1995), *Strategic Alliances: An Entrepreneurial Approach to Globalization*, Cambridge, Harvard Business Press.

Zander, U. and Kogut, B. (1995). Knowledge and the speed of the transfer and imitation of organizational capabilities: an empirical test. *Organization Science*, 6, pp. 76–92.

In: Knowledge Transfer: Practices, Types and Challenges
Editor: Dragan Ilic
ISBN: 978-1-62081-538-0

Chapter 3

CHALLENGES AND OPPORTUNITIES IN KNOWLEDGE TRANSFER BY INFORMAL AND FORMAL KNOWLEDGE BROKERS THAT SUPPORT PERSONS WITH CHRONIC PAIN

Lynn Shaw*[1]*, *Joy MacDermid*[2], *Lubna Daraz*[3] and *Bill Chedore

[1]School of Occupational Therapy, Faculty of Health Sciences, The University of Western Ontario, London, Ontario Canada

[2]School of Rehabilitation Science, McMaster University, Hamilton, Ontario, Canada

[3]Dept.of Psychiatry and Behavioural Neuroscience. McMaster University, Hamilton, Ontario, Canada

ABSTRACT

Knowledge brokers such as health care professionals and consumer group peer support leaders experience many challenges in transferring and exchanging knowledge for persons with chronic pain and those with work injuries. Meeting the needs of end users and their preferences for considering and integrating knowledge into decision making is not easy.

This chapter will provide an overview of the barriers to KT and offer strategies to facilitate ways to meet the needs of end users such as persons with chronic pain that is also sensitive to the contextual and social cultural expectations of the end users. Readers will be introduced to an Interactive Knowledge Transfer Process that can enable formal and informal knowledge brokers to create spaces and opportunities for practical knowledge exchange of research, procedural and health information needed to manage daily and work activities while living with pain.

This chapter will also have a focus on what knowledge brokers need to know to help end users successfully appraise information available on the internet.

* Corresponding author: E-mail: leshaw@uwo.ca

INTRODUCTION

Knowledge translation is a complex iterative process that involves implementing high quality evidence into action with the ultimate goal of achieving better health and participation outcomes. It often involves social processes and challenges that relate the availability and feasibility of implementing the evidence; as well as issues with the stakeholders involved in the process.

Knowledge brokers are individuals who may help bridge the gap between the source of the information; and the targets who must implement it. Knowledge brokers such as health care professionals and peer support group leaders experience many challenges in transferring and exchanging knowledge with persons who have chronic pain and work injuries.

These groups share complex needs in terms of their health issues, access to effective health care services, navigation of complex healthcare and social services that are complicated by deficiencies in high quality specific accessible information that directly relate to their needs. Meeting the needs of end users and their preferences for considering and integrating knowledge into decision making is not easy. This chapter will provide an overview of the barriers to knowledge transfer (KT) and offer strategies to facilitate meeting the needs of persons with chronic pain in a way that is sensitive to the contextual and social cultural expectations of these end users. Readers will be introduced to an Interactive Knowledge Transfer Process and three principles of KT that can enable formal and informal knowledge brokers to create spaces and opportunities for practical knowledge exchange of research, procedural, and health information needed to assist users to manage daily and work activities while living with pain. This chapter will also have a focus on what knowledge brokers need to know to help end users successfully appraise information available on the internet. Formative and informative ways to evaluate and improve ways to enhance KT by knowledge brokers will be included. Three vignettes are proposed to support how the Interactive Knowledge Transfer Process and three knowledge transfer principles might be used. One will provide an example for use by consumer peer support leaders (informal knowledge brokers) one will be for health care providers (formal knowledge brokers) and the other will be for both informal and formal knowledge brokers relevant to helping end users appraise information on the internet.

1. THE NEED FOR ACCESS TO INFORMATION AND USE OF KNOWLEDGE BROKERS

The challenge for many persons, who acquire a work injury or experience changes in functioning because of chronic pain is accessing information that can help them make informed decisions, or assisting them in understanding their current and future needs. Accessing and using knowledge is critical for persons with chronic pain to become informed about their health status (Crooks, 2006), as well as their rights and accountabilities in return to functioning, accessing services and supports, and their rights in returning to work (Shaw and Lindsay, 2008). However, the information that persons with chronic pain need to make decisions about the episodic nature of their injury or illness, understand their responsibilities for reporting and documentation, manoeuvre through the claims management process, and interact with health care professionals in the recovery and return to work processes, is often new and complex (Shaw, Knott et al. 2009; Shaw et al. 2010). For most, it is a very daunting experience to try and find information on this full spectrum of issues, let alone understand or apply relevant information to help them through their experience.

Most often persons with chronic pain look to health and rehabilitation professionals and providers in the social service sector for information or to assist them in interpreting information relevant to living and working with a disability (Shaw, MacAhonic, et al. 2009; Shaw et al. 2010). However, gaining access to the right information from the right person at the right time is not as easy or as accessible as it should be (Shaw, Knott et al, 2009; Daraz, 2011). For instance, Daraz (2011) found that women living with fibromyalgia had high information needs and preferred to receive information from healthcare providers Others have demonstrated that families members express similar needs for information (Soderberg, Strand, Haapala, Lundman, 2003). However, in their experiences healthcare providers were commonly not providing useful information. Conversely, despite concerns about quality many of these women relied on support groups and the Internet to access relevant information.

A similar trend is evident in many workers with injuries and persons with other types of chronic pain who report that they turn to disability, pain or injured worker groups to gain access to the information and knowledge needed to make sense of the new and often challenging processes they encounter in finding their way back to work (Shaw, MacAhonic et al. 2009, Shaw, MacDemid et al. 2010). This extended search for information suggests that there are a number of informal knowledge brokers that persons with chronic pain and disabilities seek out.

It is evident that injured workers and patients with chronic pain who encounter a lack of understanding of their needs actively seek out people who share their experiences as a potential source of relevant information. This barrier to accessing information suggests that the role of knowledge broker might be an optimal knowledge translation strategy. Shaw, the first author of this paper defines *Knowledge Brokers* as people who offer access and insights into the relevance and meaning of information to facilitate understanding, help a person adapt and / or to begin to change ways of being and doing in daily, health and work life. Knowledge brokers are sometimes classified as formal or informal. This division is related to the context whereby the knowledge broker assumes the role – not the quality of the information or success of the strategy. Formal knowledge brokers include health care professionals where there is a presumption they have been trained with relevant knowledge and associated communication skills (Booth, 2011). This group would also include individuals with specific training in contextualizing appropriate information for target audiences that are hired to perform the role of broker knowledge. Informal knowledge brokers are those with experiential expertise that share it through support groups or consumer run agencies. Knowledge brokers can be formal, i.e. health care professionals or specific champions hired to broker knowledge or information, where as informal knowledge brokers are those with experiential expertise and share it through support groups or consumer run agencies. Research suggests that persons with chronic pain experience barriers in accessing information but also that the formal (healthcare professionals) and informal knowledge brokers (support groups) find it challenging to meet the realm of information needs of persons with chronic pain (Shaw, MacAhonic et al. 2009; Shaw, Knott et al. 2009; Shaw, Pye and Dodman 2009; Shaw, MacDermid et al, 2010). In this chapter we will address system and practice challenges.

Strategies will emphasize processes that formal and informal knowledge brokers can use to enhance and improve knowledge transfer efforts, including use the internet, to meet the needs of end-users – persons with chronic pain and work injuries. Ways to evaluate the strategies used to support knowledge transfer and uptake by end-users will also be provided for consideration in continuous attention to adopt strategies that work.

2. Some of the System Challenges and Barriers

A series of research studies looking at system barriers that prevent the full participation of persons with disabilities in the service and care processes unveiled that access to knowledge and information is a major gap in the lived experiences of persons with disabilities (Korzycki et al., 2008; Shaw, Leyshon and Lui, 2007; Shaw, MacKinnon, et al., 2004; Shaw, McWilliam, et al., 2007; Shaw, Sumsion, et al., 2004). This problem in accessing information is consistent with the findings of others (Friesen et al., 2001; MacDermid et al., 2008). More recently, research studies on system barriers to return to work have consistently identified the need for greater access to information for persons with work injuries and chronic pain: Roberts-Yates (2003) suggested that accessibility to information is a key area for research; Pohlman et al. (2001) advocated for standard terminology to foster shared understandings; and Baril et al. (2003) and Friesen et al. (2001) similarly stress that in Canada there is a need to build better supports and trust in communications across all stakeholders in the return to work process. In the area of participatory ergonomics, Loisel et al. (2001) also demonstrated the effect of involving workers in the collaborative process in workplace change to improve safety and prevent disability. Beyond this Farkas and Anthony in the United States (2007) identified that there is a gap in knowledge transfer in that 'what is known' is not necessarily or consistently influencing 'what is done' in practice or policies. They suggest that rehabilitation research centers need to take an active role in promoting dissemination, utilization and evaluation of knowledge transfer processes. Shaw and colleagues (Shaw, MacAhonic et al. 2009 and Shaw, MacDermid et al. 2010) also noted that the engagement of chronic pain and worker support group representatives in the research process is missing yet their input is needed to inform best practice in knowledge transfer with injured workers who have chronic pain. Some of the barriers to accessing information are related to the unfamiliarity with the process of navigating the complex systems of expectations across health, social and workplace services (Shaw, MacDermid et al. 2010). For persons with chronic pain they lack access to appropriate outpatient care or services especially when they are no longer work attached or are unemployed (Shaw, Pye and Dodman, 2009). Information on the web is often contradictory as well as health care providers often have different views on best practices for chronic pain that adds to confusion and skepticism (Shaw, MacDermid et al. 2010). There is a lack of dedicated services and resources for persons with chronic pain. Furthermore there is no integration of services and communications among knowledge brokers – formal and informal or across sectors such as health and social care providers (Shaw, MacDermid et al. 2010). Underscoring these challenges is the absence of evidenced informed policy to direct funding for chronic pain services. Given the realm of these barriers and challenges there is a need for a process to sustain collaboration with chronic pain and worker support groups in brokering knowledge to ensure that the needs of persons with chronic pain are considered in the research process.

Knowledge translation is an emerging field where theories and strategies are evolving. To date, most of the emphasis on knowledge exchange and transfer (KET) has focused on knowledge transfer between researchers and clinicians (Shaw, 2011) or policy–makers (see this site for an example of how knowledge brokers influence policy makers http://www.cihr-irsc.gc.ca/e/30673.html). This trend is fuelled by the need for using evidence-based approaches in health care (Ho et al., 2004). There is a growing trend however, to include the public in the knowledge exchange and translation process related to health research by the Canadian Institute for Health Research. Typically these groups focus on a targeted health or disease. A recent article by Shea and colleagues (2005) describes a collaborative process for engaging consumers in partnerships. Their aims were to achieve wide participation of stakeholders, including consumers, to guide research and its dissemination through the Cochrane Musculoskeletal Group (CMSG). The experience of the CMSG underscores the need for relationship building and promoting team responsibilities for consumers. More recently Shaw (2011) calls for more immediate change in knowledge transfer and that is to focus on what end-users need and want. She calls for the field of work rehabilitation to adopt a strategic plan to promote knowledge transfer for end-users and this be a priority for academics, clinicians, stakeholders and informal support group knowledge brokers and educators.

3. Challenges in Knowledge Brokering

Challenges in meeting the needs of persons with chronic pain were studied by Shaw and colleagues (2010). Findings from consultations, focus groups and interviews with 63 Injured worker group representatives, 43 health care professionals and 2 professional knowledge brokers (representing 3 organizations) identified the following barriers (see Figure 1) they faced in helping persons with work injuries and chronic pain access and use the information they need:

- Lack of accessible information in diverse formats and locations
- Lack of consistent knowledge exchange between health and social service professionals as well as between health professionals and worker's support groups
- Lack of appreciation of the depth of consumer informational needs
- Lack of consistent views by some health care professionals about their role in knowledge transfer with persons with chronic pain and work injuries
- Lack of time with health care providers to explore if the information retrieved on the web is relevant or useful
- Lack of consistent views about sourcing information, and what formats are considered best practice
- Lack of healthcare professional understanding of a worker or person with chronic pain capacity and readiness to use information
- Lack of a common knowledge translation guide for health professionals and worker support groups.

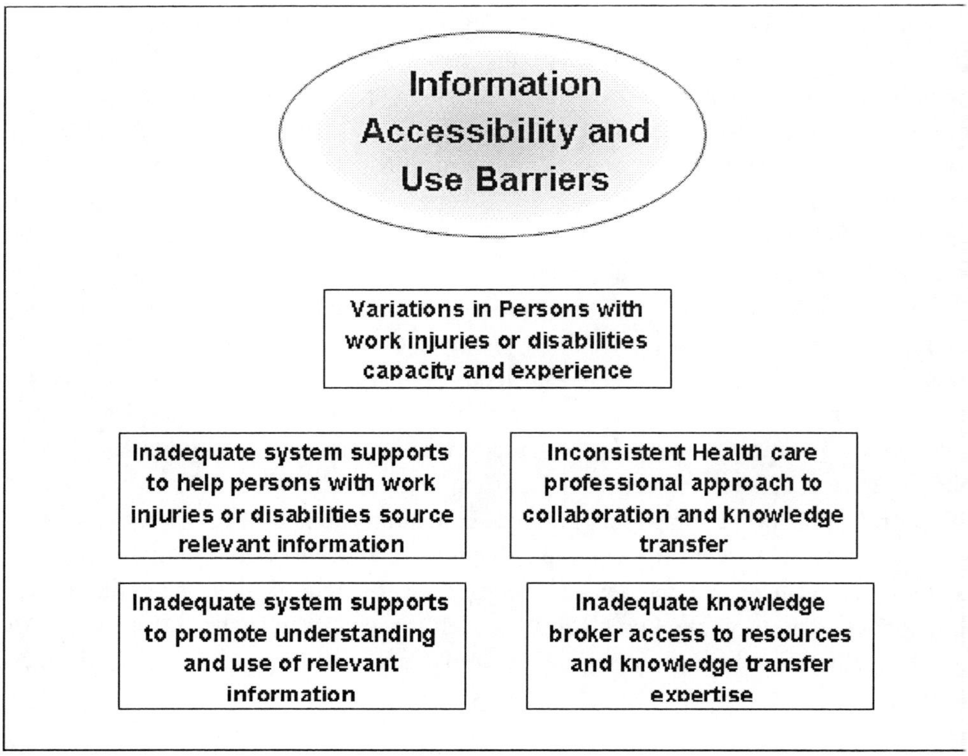

Figure 1. Barriers and challenges to information use and access. Adapted from Shaw, MacDermid et al. 2010.

Likewise Shaw and others (Shaw, Pye and Dodman, 2009) identified in a study with persons with chronic pain and work injuries that access to information was a problem but that it was also underscored by a lack of transparency, and trust. This culminated in persons with work injuries and chronic pain becoming skeptical of information and discarding rather than considering information or sources as credible.

Lack of simplification of information or diverse formats precluded understanding, and a lack of support for considering the relevance of information made it difficult to act on or adapt or redesign health management strategies or redesign lifestyles to live or adjust to the episodic nature of chronic pain (Shaw, Pye and Dodman, 2009).

4. Knowledge Broker Development of Skills

The successful knowledge broker has a unique set of skills that make able to perform complex processes that initiate change through use of information. These skills were described by Lomas (2007) and include: Entrepreneurial (networking, problem solving, innovating), trusted and credible, clear communicator, understands the cultures of both the research and decision making environments, able to find and assess relevant research in a variety of formats, facilitates, mediates, and negotiates and understands the principles of adult learning. This set of skills indicates why either formal or informal knowledge brokers might be most effective in different situations. While clinicians may have training in adult learning, and how to access research evidence they may be less knowledgeable about the culture of the knowledge users and may have limited training on how to target the social channels of their targets. The converse is often true of the informal knowledge broker. For example, for injured workers the experience of having to deal with navigating the complex regulations/responsibilities of workers compensation, changes in their occupational roles, interpersonal relationships while managing the ongoing issues with their health problem can be overwhelming (Shaw, MacAhonic et al. 2009; Shaw, MacDermid et al, 2010). Clinicians often provide help with the health care issues; but rarely meet the other needs often filled by informal knowledge brokers. Neither type of knowledge broker has the complete set of skills required; nor is formal training typically available. Knowledge brokers often immerse themselves in different environments; and access others performing the same role (see for more information on knowledge brokers, http://www.knowledgebrokersforum.org/219319) to enhance their effectiveness. This process continues to perpetuate the separation of formal and informal knowledge brokers. More efforts are needed to interact and learn form each other and to draw on the strengths to support a more integrated approach to support the needs of end-users.

5. What are the Information Needs with Chronic Pain and Work Injuries

The realm of information needs that persons with chronic pain are reported extensively in the literature. For instance, Shaw, MacAhonic et al, (2007) and MacAhonic (2006) identified that injured workers with chronic conditions require 8 dimensions of information and supports. Information and knowledge needs included informational supports, emotional supports, advocacy supports, instrumental supports, transformation supports, lobbying supports, appraisal and evaluation supports and community of practice supports (See Figure 2). A scoping review on episodic illness and chronic pain by Antao et al. also revealed fears of workers further suggest the types of information that persons with chronic pain and intermittent work capacity need (Antao et al. in press).

Information is needed to address the fear of losing health insurance coverage/benefits, fear of managing finances, fear of loss of financial support (both long term sick leave benefits and drug plans), financially supporting children, childcare needs, costs for medications, and other general financial issues.

Further to this, Shaw, et al. (2010) found that formal and informal knowledge brokers did not encounter requests for research based information from persons with chronic pain and work injuries rather they would accept research based information if it was provided by a health care professional.

Persons with chronic pain had more targeted needs for information. For instance, Daraz et al. (2011) studied the informational needs of 442 women with fibromyalgia and found that the top 5 most important information needs were treatment options, impacts on daily life, how to cope with fibromyalgia, impact on work ability and changes to my health. Daraz explored the information preferences of these women and found that websites and online sources were the most frequently used sources followed by support groups, people with the same conditions, a doctor and health care providers.

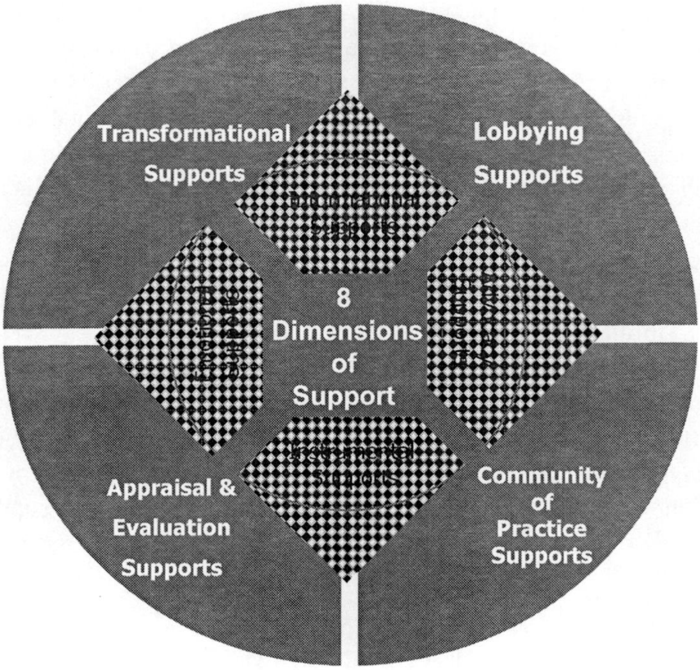

Figure 2. 8 Dimensions of Support Model, Graphically conceptualized by MacAhonic and Shaw, 2007 and published in Work 2009 see Shaw, MacAhonic, et al. 2009.

To address these barriers and to overcome the difficulties that knowledge brokers experience in making sure that they can meet a range of informational needs Shaw, MacDermid et al. (2010) recommended that best practice guides for KT be developed for health care professionals and members of support groups. Strategies that can be used by knowledge brokers need to consider ways to over come the specific barriers and challenges and to adopt strategies to Facilitate Interactive Knowledge Transfer as outlined by Shaw and colleagues (See Figure 3).

There are six main strategies that knowledge brokers can use:1. Understand the person's or worker's context and readiness, 2. Explore and determine information needs, 3. Engage the person in information exchange, 4. Include time and develop a plan for regular opportunities for KT, 5. Develop a social context and identify other contexts to promote KT, 6.Tailor information (match approach with needs of person). The strategies are organized in Figure 3 to represent the interactive nature of the processes between the knowledge brokers and persons with chronic pain or work injuries.

These strategies were organized and displayed in separate ellipses in Figure 3 and do not assume any specific order. Shaw and colleagues also found knowledge brokers make conscious efforts to prepare themselves to support the knowledge transfer process through staying abreast of new information and/or sourcing information on the internet or through networking (Shaw, MacDermid et al, 2010). These actions occurred in the background and are represented in Figure 3 by the grey circle that joins them together.

In addition, persons with chronic pain and work injuries also concurred with these findings in that they identified that they need others to help create safe spaces for KT and support for seeking and searching for information (Shaw, MacDermid et al, 2010).

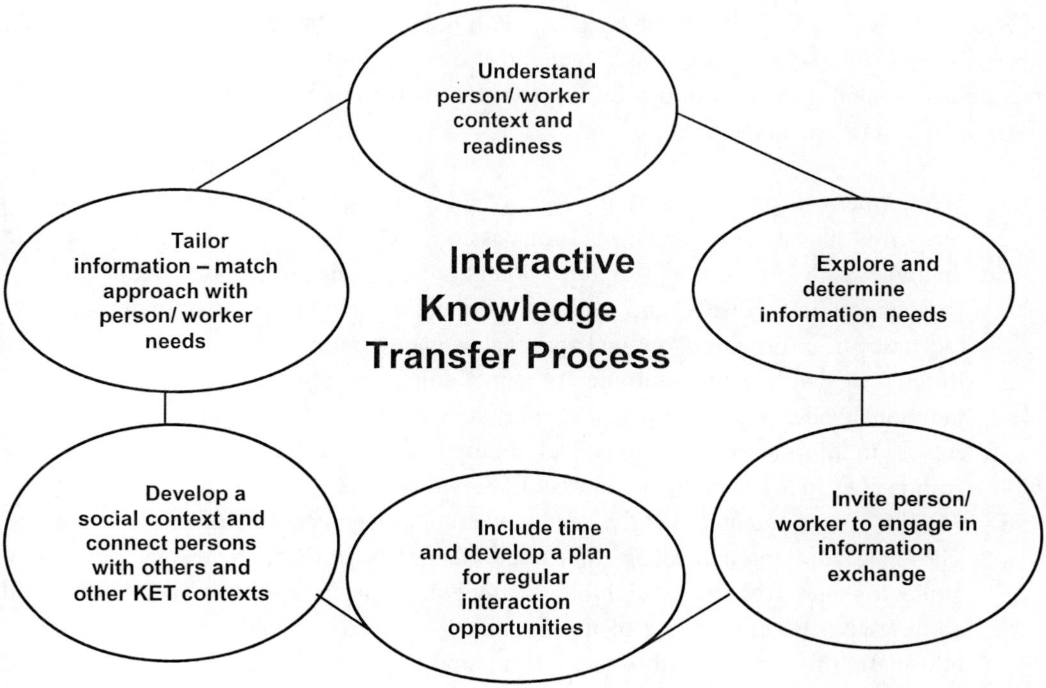

Figure 3. Facilitators of an Interactive Knowledge Transfer Process. Adapted from Shaw, MacDermid et al. 2010.

Strategies that persons with chronic pain suggest are needed to promote avenues for personal change when living with newly exposed and long term disabilities include opportunities for appraising the self in context, taking time to reflect and learn about new information and to include a focus on planning for contingencies due to the long term nature and intermittent work capacity associated with chronic pain (Shaw, Pye and Dodman, 2009). Shaw and her colleagues (2009) also posited that three key principles of 1) equitable access through fairness and transparency, 2) understanding through simplification and participation, and 3) interpretation, use, and action through interaction, reflection and integration need to be built into the approaches that knowledge brokers use to transfer information see Figure 4.

All of these facilitators, strategies and principles underscored the need to develop a template for informal and formal knowledge brokers to use to improve their efforts in KT to meet the needs of end-users, persons with chronic pain and work injuries.

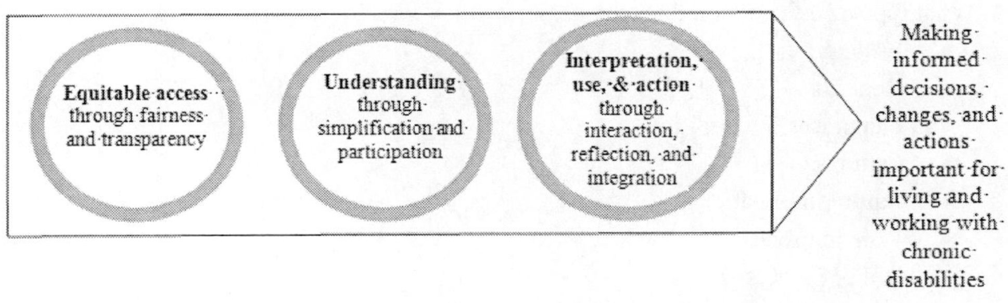

Figure 4. Principles of KT for persons with chronic pain that support knowledge use. Adapted from Shaw et al. 2009 CJOT.

See Figure 5 for a knowledge broker template in working with persons with chronic pain who have work injuries or work disabilities and want to return to function and work. This template is based on five assumptions for KT for persons with chronic pain and work injuries developed by Shaw and colleagues:

1. Worker/person participation and involvement in KT is important and can be supported through, dialogue and discussion, ongoing learning, interacting and dialogue with others that supports validation, learning and uptake, reflecting on information individually and with others, and developing shared understandings (accuracy of information, optimal approaches in communication);
2. Return to work and returning to functioning are highly contextualized and individualized processes, but also supported by common set of rights;
3. Access to information is not universal, requires diversity;
4. Approaches to KT need to be tailored to individual; and
5. Support is fundamental to early, accurate and ongoing access to information sources. These assumptions underscore the proposed best practice strategies can serve as a guide to support knowledge brokers in helping persons with work injuries and chronic pain become aware of information they need, understand the relevance of information they want, and to use information important to them to make informed decisions.

A. Understand worker context and readiness to receive, use, understand, share and exchange.

Consider:

- Educational level, literacy skills, language barriers, comfort level with research and information
- Mental health status, anxiety, ability to retain information
- Ability to take in information – affected by diagnosis, readiness and relationships
- Understand current 'filters' how the person/worker sees or perceives information – what lens and criteria is the person using
- Cultural issues that support information use – meaning of illness, role of family, inter vs. intra dependent, environment

B. Explore and determine what type of information the person/worker needs and want to do with knowledge and information.

Consider:

1. What type of information does the person/worker want or need.
    - Process
    - Benefits
    - Diagnoses or condition
    - Options
    - Future implications
    - Role in process
    - Role of others
    - Time lines
    - Other

---

2. What does the person/worker want to do with information –

- Apply it to their injury or condition,
- Learn about the process
- Understand the relevance to current situation
- Compare it to other information
- Make decisions
- Act on information to use information for understand
- Help others understand
- Understand the short term and long consequences
- Other

C. Invite person/worker to engage in information exchange

Consider:

- Develop shared expectations for information exchange
- Honour independence
- Suggest ideas
- Provide choice
- Encourage reflection – thinking about relevance of information to personal situation
- Provide insights into how information can be used – explore pros and cons
- Other

D. Include time and develop a plan for regular opportunities to: check understanding, developed shared understanding, address misperceptions, and invite discussion on emerging or new insights and information.

Move person from awareness to understanding and to integration to become confident in decision-making – using knowledge critically and applying it in an informed way to make decisions or to change or to adapt or redesign health and work lifestyle.

Consider:

- Focus on factual information
- Focus on reflection to identify meaningful information
- Use examples to promote interpretation
- Use examples to promote skills in applying knowledge to make decisions
- Engage groups of persons in sharing experiences in using information and finding information
- Encourage discussion with family members or friends
- Build time into programs for knowledge sharing and reflection these processes to occur.
- Other

E. Develop a social context and identify other contexts that support knowledge and information exchange that welcomes and invites person/worker involvement and partnership in KT as a central part of the process of getting better, finding their way through the process of healing, returning to work, managing while at work, trying to return to function and participation in everyday life.

Figure 5. Continued on next page.

Consider:

- Safety
- Comfort
- Confidentiality
- Convey confidence and reassurance
- Need for learning
- Need for validation
- Need for ongoing learning, support, education, connection
- Other

F. Tailor information – match approach with IW needs

Consider and develop:

- Different formats – verbal; written text; internet; pictures; props; analogies
- Use plain language guidelines for text and plain language in audio form
- Different language translations
- The more complex the issue the more formats should be used – to support multimodal learning
- Use art and story telling (not necessarily therapy); didactic sharing and learning opportunities; conversational; peer contact
- Establish call-in centre for impromptu needs
- Provide research information in functional language and use everyday examples
- Simplify/break down information
- Prioritize informational needs
- Other

Figure 5. Template for knowledge brokers to support an Interactive Knowledge Transfer Process (developed by Shaw, L., MacDermid, J., Kothari, A., Duncan, A., Lindsay, R., Brake, P., Page, P., Argyle, C., March, 2008).

6. Other Supports that Knowledge Brokers Need

Knowledge brokers need supports to be as effective as they can in didactic and group interactions with persons with chronic pain. Thus the needs of knowledge brokers themselves must also be considered. Knowledge brokers need both the time and resources to effectively broker knowledge (Ward, House Hamer, 2009). In addition, they need access to supportive materials that can assist them to synthesize information, identify credible e-sites and information, and also help them help persons/workers evaluate the credibility of information sources as well as learn methods on how to source information (Daraz et l, 2011; Shaw, MacDermid et al. 2010; Dobbins et al, 2009). Dobbins and colleagues also identified that formal knowledge brokers need to be able to tailor messages, gather evidence, critically appraise, synthesize and interpret what evidence means in the big picture. Thus, they need system supports and funding to be able to become as effective as possible. Knowledge brokers also need to access policy makers be able to develop trusting relationships to foster knowledge transfer (Dobbins, et al, 2009). Given these requirements knowledge brokers also need education on KT approaches or models as well as what time to fully understand the culture, context and the supports and services exist in local areas. It is key for formal and informal knowledge brokers to become aware of the realm of supports that are available and to work collaboratively towards meeting the needs of end-users. Finally, there is a strong need to evaluate KT efforts and to know what strategies are working and to assess the ongoing needs and preferences of persons with chronic pain and work injuries (Shaw, MacDermid et al. 2010).

7. ACCESSING AND USING THE INTERNET SOURCES

There exist more than 70,000 websites that offer health information (Stats Canada, [1] for consumers. Many of these sites are accessed by people with fibromyalgia as the internet has become a major source for information for them (Fox and Rainie, 2009; Daraz et al, 2011). About 92% of people with fibromyalgia believe that online information is useful for them and the majority of them frequently use the Internet to access information about fibromyalgia (Daraz et al. 2011).

This immense use of websites is due to their desire to understand their health condition and its prognosis, treatment options, disease management strategies, and to make informed decisions about their health. People with fibromyalgia also want to know potential symptoms, diagnosis, medications, exercise, diet/food, alternative therapies, specialists, coping strategies, changes in health, changes in life style, support groups, new research, and self-management so that they are able to understand the consequences of the disease (Fox and Rainie , 2009; Daraz, 2011).

On the other hand, people have concerns about the difficult use of medical terminology and lack of quality of online health information. They prefer to have information given by healthcare providers and other reputable sources in a simple and usable format. In addition, people with fibromyalgia want to have information about fibromyalgia combined in a package that is up-to-date, relevant, consistent, accurate, easy to read and easy to access (Fox and Rainie , 2009; Daraz, 2011).

Interest in searching the web for health information is growing which is indicated by high and increasing usage by consumers. In Canada about 8.7 million people (Stats Canada) and in the USA, about 61% people (Fox and Rainie, 2009) access the Internet to obtain medical and health-related information. However, concerns remain about the use of online health information for health matters. Some information on the web can be highly authoritative, some can be strong community appeal, but much can also be of questionable quality.

Low quality information can be harmful for health if used inappropriately by consumers. While information is critical to living with chronic illnesses, existing information resources are unlikely to provide necessary or accurate information and may not be usable for people in terms of answering their questions and satisfying their needs.

Consumers tend to be non-clinical and may not be able to assess the quality of online health information. Yet, many consumers who go online to access health information expressed the need for evidence-based information. For example, a qualitative study by Daraz demonstrated that women with Fibromyalgia have difficulty in understanding the medical or technical languages used on websites to put the information into context (Daraz, 2011).

Majority of the information they were able to find online were inconsistent, not reliable, contradictory, and out-of-dated. It is therefore, important for knowledge brokers to recognize and assess the potential harms and benefits of online health information. To address the concerns of quality of online health information, many organizations and individuals have published web health assessment tools and guidelines.

8. Evaluating Internet Resources Tools for Knowledge Brokers

There are almost 151 tools available which include 125 websites and 26 articles to help consumers evaluate the quality of online information (see Health Improvement Institute website). Daraz and others performed a systematic analysis to evaluate four major tools developed by well-known organizations (Daraz, MacDermid, Wilkins, and Shaw, 2009). These tools were: AMA guidelines, HON Code of Conduct, Medline Plus guideline and Health Promotion instrument.

Their review demonstrated that these tools did not meet the literacy level and ease of use for general consumers. There is another well-known tool available called the DISCERN which has been used by many to evaluate publication reliability and quality of information on treatment choices (Charnock, Shepperd, Needham, and Gann, (1999).

However, DISCERN does not allow a person the ability to assess many of the important criteria that are important for assessing the content of specific information and for the development and dissemination process to distribute information, for example, accuracy, completeness, disclosure and readability (Eysenbach, and Kohler, 2002).

ITEMS TOPIC	ITEMS SUB-TOPIC	QUALITY CHECKLIST
Authorship	Advice given by qualified Professionals	1. Is the author of the information clearly identified?
		2. Can you tell if qualified professionals are giving the advice?
Content	Quality	3. Does it appear that the topic is well covered?
		4. Does the web site provide clear reference of sources of information (includes scientific studies)?
Currency	Date of publication	5. Does the information indicate the date of publication?
Usefulness	Appropriate for target audience	6. Do you find the information usable and understandable?
Disclosure	Identify funding source	7. Can you tell who owns this website?
		8. Does the website identify its funding source?
User Support	Contact address for author/editor	9. Is there any contact information provided?
Privacy and Confidentiality	Respect privacy and confidentiality of visitors	10. Can you use the website anonymously?

Figure 6. Checklist to assess the quality of online health information. (Adapted from: Daraz et al. 2009).

Daraz and others developed a tool based on their analysis of existing quality tools and agreed that a comprehensive evaluation of website contents should consider the following criteria: authorship, content, currency, usefulness, disclosure, user support, privacy and confidentiality (Daraz, MacDermid, Wilkins, and Shaw, 2009).

In addition to these criteria evaluation of reading level for general consumer use of online health information is also important. Anyone who aims to provide health information should try to achieve a grade level of 6 to 8 to achieve literacy levels for general consumers. For reading level evaluation, "The Flesch-Kincaid Grade Level" formula can be used (see the document The Flesch Reading Ease website).

Vignette #1: If you are a formal knowledge broker such as a health care professional what would you advise a person with chronic pain due to fibromyalgia when searching the internet?. Consider criteria of author credibility, content accuracy, currency of information, the disclosure of where the information came from and who generated the information.

8. Evaluation of KT processes

Many research granting agencies are concerned with knowledge dissemination and the transfer mechanisms used to share the results of research findings. More recently granting agencies are requiring that research proposals include budget allocation and approaches for KT. For the most part, the examination of the effectiveness of KT extends to end-users in the health sector such as professionals or policy/decision makers in health contexts. The challenge for the knowledge broker is twofold. One is to evaluate their effectiveness in transferring information and to evaluate the effectiveness of the approaches used transfer knowledge that is used to support change or adaption of the end-users.

Thus there are formative evaluation approaches that have been developed to examine outcomes of KT. For instance, Dobbins et al. (2009) have examined the effectiveness of knowledge brokering. Another example is by Skinner (2007) who developed a measure to examine in-depth the dimensions of *reach* and *uptake* in the use of KT strategies.

Reach refers to how many people does the information extend to or actually access new knowledge and uptake refers to the degree to which it is considered or used. Others have used formal approaches such as examining commitment to change (Mazmanian et al. 1999) immediately post KT sessions at subsequent intervals. However, other mechanisms are needed to evaluate the utility of the knowledge and the potential for changing professional practices and approaches in provision of service or care or interventions. Furthermore, approaches are needed to assess the relevance of knowledge for other end-users.

To date, many of these formal evaluation approaches have not been applied to end-users such as persons with pain. If end-users such as health care consumers are involved in more integrated KT approaches (Graham, et al. 2006) then evaluation will be more focused on evidence-based health knowledge. Very few evaluations of KT extend to procedural or knowledge of coping strategies needed to live and work with a chronic disability. Other informal approaches such as focus groups to elicit feedback might be considered and formal approaches such as pre and post survey KT sessions to gain insights into the utilization of information. For persons with chronic pain areas for evaluation need to be consistent and coherent with key concepts outlined by Shaw, Pye and Dodman (2007) that focus on *reach* -

the equitable access to information (transparent and inclusive), and to what extent do the mechanisms support *uptake* - an understanding of the information, support interaction, integration and reflection to consider relevance and potential applicability of knowledge to promote change or adaptation. Knowledge brokers need to consider the use of evaluative formats to enable KT at both the group and individual level.

Vignette #2 If you are an informal knowledge broker who runs support groups what formal or informal evaluation method is appropriate for understanding the use of interactive approaches on knowledge use by persons with chronic pain that attend face to face groups or online groups.

Consider: The use of integrating time in groups to explore what knowledge or information they used from previous group sessions and if they passed on information to others. Build on this by asking for input on what information they need more of and what formats work best.

Vignette #3: If you are a formal knowledge broker working one-on-one with clients or patients with chronic pain what formal evaluation method might you use to evaluate uptake?

Consider: The use of a commitment to change form ask them to note the specific knowledge they found useful and to create an action plan to do something new or different as a result of the knowledge. Next follow up and review in a month to find out how they used knowledge to make an adjustment or do something differently. Keep a record of the number of people that committed to change and then enacted change..

Conclusion

Knowledge broker capacity, skills and resources are essential for getting the right knowledge into the hands of end-users so that information can be used toward change. Knowledge brokers can develop best practices in KT by creating milieus for KT that can foster reflection and use of knowledge for persons with chronic pain and work injuries. Knowledge use can serve to empower and lead to self-management needed to live and work with chronic pain.

References

Antao, L., Shaw, L., Ollson, K., Reen, K., To, F. Bossers, A., Cooper, L. Chronic Pain and episodic illness and its effects on occupation. WORK (in press).

Baril, R., Clarke, J., Friesen, M., Stock, S., Cole, D., and the Work-Ready group. (2003). Management of return-to-work programs for workers with musculoskeletal disorders: A qualitative study in three Canadian provinces. *Social Science and Medicine, 57,* 2101-2114.

Booth A. Bridging the 'Know-Do Gap': a role for health information professionals? *Health Info Libr J* 2011 December;28(4):331-334.

Canadian Population Health Initiative. (2001, February). *An environmental scan of research transfer strategies.* Ottawa, ON: Canadian Institute for Health Information.

Charnock, D., Shepperd, S., Needham, G., and Gann, R. (1999). DISCERN: An instrument for judging the quality of written consumer health information on treatment choices. *Journal of Epidemiology and Community Health*, *53*,105–111.

Crooks VA. I go on the Internet; I always, you know, check to see what's new" chronically ill women's use of online health information to shape and inform doctor patient interactions in the space of care provision. *ACME: An Intern E-Journal for Crit Geograp* 2006;5:50-69.

Daraz L, MacDermid JC, Wilkins S, Gibson J, and Shaw L. Information preferences of people living with Fibromyalgia – a survey of their information needs and preferences. *Rheumatology Reports*. 2011, Volume 3 (1).

Daraz, L. "Information availability and needs of people living with fibromyalgia" (January 1, 2011). ETD Collection for McMaster University. Paper AAINR74587. URL. http://digitalcommons.mcmaster.ca/dissertations/AAINR74587

Daraz, L., MacDermid, J. C., Wilkins, S., and Shaw, L. (2009). Tools to evaluate the quality of web health information. *The International Journal of Technology, Knowledge and Society,* 5 (3), 127-142.

Dobbins, M., Robeson P., Ciliska, D., Hanna, S., Cameron, R., O'Mara, L. and Mercer S. A description of a knowledge broker role implemented as part of a randomized controlled trial evaluating three knowledge translation strategies. *Implementation Science* 2009, 4:23 doi:10.1186/1748-5908-4-23.

Eysenbach, G., and Kohler, C. (2002). How do consumers search for and appraise health information on the World Wide Web? Qualitative study using focus groups, usability tests, and in-depth interviews. *BMJ, 324*, 573-577.

Friesen, M., Yassi, A., and Cooper, J. (2001). Return-to-work: The importance of human interactions and organizational structures. *Work, 17,* 11-22.

Graham, I.D, Logan, J, Harrison, M, Straus, S., Tetroe, J., Caswell, W., Robinson, N. (2006) Lost in Knowledge Translation: Time for a Map? *The Journal of Continuing Education in the Health Professions*, Volume 26, pp. 13–24.

Grandinetti DA. Doctors and the web: Help your patients surf the Net safely. *Med Econ* 2000;77:186e8.

Health Improvement Institute. A Report on the Evaluation of Criteria Sets for Assessing Health Web Sites. [Online Document] URL http://www.hii.org/index.html.

Ho, K., Bloch, R., Gondocz, T., Laprise, R., Perrier, L, Ryan, D., et al. (2004). Technology-enabled knowledge translation: Frameworks to promote research and practice. *Journal of Continuing Education in the Health Professions, 24,* 90-99.

Korzycki, M., Korzycki, M., and Shaw, L. (2008). Left behind in the return-to work journey: Consumer insights for policy change and practice strategies. *WORK.*

Lomas, J. (2007). The in-between world of knowledge brokering. *BMJ,* 334, 129-132.

MacAhonic, P. (2006) Feasibility study for BC injured workers Centre. Unpublished Masters of Business Administration Thesis. Royal Roads University.

MacDermid, J., Geldart, S., Williams, R., Westmorland, M., Lin, C., and Shannon, H. (2008). Work Organization and Health: A qualitative study of the perceptions of workers. *WORK*, 30 (3) 241-254.

Mazmanian, P.E., Mazmanian, P.M. (1999). Commitment to change: Theoretical foundations, methods, and outcomes. *Journal of Continuing Education in the Health Professions*. Volume 19, Issue 4, 200–207.

Pohlman, J., Poosawtsee, C., Gerndt, K., and Lindstrom-Hazel, D. (2001). Improving work programs' delivery of information and service to workers' compensation carriers. *Work, 16,* 91-100.

Roberts-Yates, C. (2003). The concerns and issues of injured workers in relation to claims/injury management and rehabilitation: The need for new operational frameworks. *Disability and Rehabilitation, 25,* 898-907.

Shaw, L. (2011). Knowledge transfer in work practice: Challenging the status quo to meet the needs of end users. *WORK*, 40, (3) 337-341.

Shaw, L., and Lindsay, R. Renewing focus and building capacity for enacting authentic collaboration in work rehabilitation. *WORK,* 30, 215-218, 2008.

Shaw, L., Knott, M., Lindsay, R., Brake, P., Page P., Argyle, C., MacDermid, J., and Kothari, A. (2009) Opening doors to information for injured workers through knowledge exchange and research with consumer community groups. *Occupational Therapy Now*, July/August 11, 23-26.

Shaw, L., Leyshon, R., and Liu, M. (2007). Validating the potential of the ICF to elaborate barriers to and facilitators of consumer participation. Canadian Journal of Occupational Therapy, *ICF Special Issue*, 74, 255-66.

Shaw, L., MacAhonic, P., Lindsay, R. and Brake, P. (2009). Evaluating the support needs of injured workers in managing occupational transitions after injury. *WORK*, 32. (4), 477-490.

Shaw, L., MacDermid ,J., Kothari, A., Lindsay, R., Brake, P., Page, P., Argyle, C., Gagnon, C., and Knott, M. (2010). Knowledge brokering with injured workers: Perspectives of injured worker groups and health care professionals. *WORK.*, 36 (1) 89-101.

Shaw, L., MacKinnon, J., McWilliam, C. L., and Sumsion, T. (2004). Consumer participation in the employment rehabilitation process: Contextual factors and implications for practice. *Work*, *23*(3), 181-192.

Shaw, L., McWilliam, C., Sumsion, T., and MacKinnon., J. (2007). Optimizing environments for consumer participation and self-direction in finding employment. *Occupational Therapy Journal of Research, 27(2),* 59-70.

Shaw, L., Pye, K., and Dodman, J. (2009) Client insights on knowledge use and access in return to work. Canadian Journal of Occupational Therapy, 76 (5) 359-367.

Shaw, L., Sumsion, T., McWilliam, C. L, and MacKinnon, J. (2004). Service providers perspectives on including consumers in the vocational rehabilitation service process. *The Journal of Vocational Rehabilitation 21(3),* 123-136.

Shea, B., Santesso, N., Qualman, A., Heiberg, T., Leong, A., Judd, M., et al. (2005). Consumer-driven health care: Building partnerships in research. *Health Expectations, 8,* 352-359.

Soderberg S, Strand M, Haapala M, Lundman B. Living with a woman with fibromyalgia from the perspective of the husband. *J Adv Nurs* 2003 April;42(2):143-150.

Skinner (2007). Developing a tool to measure knowledge exchange outcomes. *The Canadian Journal of Program Evaluation*, 22, 49-73.

Statistics Canada. Canadian Internet Use Survey (CIUS). http://www.statcan.gc.ca/

The Flesch Reading Ease. Readability Formulas.com. Free Readability Assessment. http://www.readabilityformulas.com/free-readability-formula-assessment.php

Ward, V., House, A., and Hamer, S. (2009). Knowledge brokering: The missing link in the evidence to action chain? *Evidence Policy,* 5(3): 267–279. doi:10.1332 /174426409X463811.

In: Knowledge Transfer: Practices, Types and Challenges ISBN: 978-1-62081-538-0
Editor: Dragan Ilic

Chapter 4

Utilising Evidence Based Practice to Facilitate Knowledge Transfer

Dragan Ilic*

Department of Epidemiology and Preventive Medicine,
School of Public Health and Preventive Medicine, Monash University, VIC, Australia

Abstract

The principles of evidence based practice focus on providing users with the skills to identify, evaluate and implement evidence within a clinical setting. A similar process is also apparent with knowledge transfer, which also takes into account barriers and facilitators of evidence uptake by stakeholders. This chapter will explore how the principles of evidence based practice may be utilized by individuals to facilitate knowledge transfer from a user's perspective.

Introduction

The concept of evidence-based medicine, also referred to as evidence-based practice (EBP), was introduced in 1991 as a method for assisting health professionals with obtaining information and synthesizing its usefulness to aid clinical decision making.[1]The EBP process integrates the best available research evidence along with a health professional's clinical expertise and the values of the patient. [2]Clinical expertise draws on the health professional's clinical skills and past experience to identify and treat each patient's individual circumstance. Patient values encompass the personal concerns, expectations, cultural influences and characteristics of individuals during the clinical encounter. The best research evidence draws on the highest quality of clinically related research.

This chapter will provide a commentary on how EBP may assist with promoting knowledge transfer within the healthcare system. It will define what EBP is, how health professionals may increase their competency in it and how EBP can be used to ensure that the

---

* Corresponding author: E-mail: dragan.ilic@monash.edu

most reliable evidence is routinely implemented into medical decision making to ensure that patients receive the best care, in line with their own patient values.

Why is EBP Important?

A number of approaches can be taken when making decisions in healthcare, which include;

1) Tradition ("We've always done it this way"),
2) Convention ("Everyone else always does it this way"),
3) Belief ("I believe the natural way is best"), or
4) Evidence-based (That is based on some sort of systematic assessment of evidence). [3]

The first three methods are highly reliant on opinion, or eminence-based practice, which can be a hazardous approach to practicing healthcare. The move to be more 'evidence-based' was highlighted by Archie Cochrane, who performed a systematic review of data from seven randomized controlled trials (RCTs) comparing a course of corticosteroids, compared to placebo, given to women at risk of entering premature labour. [4]This systematic review indicated that by 1972 there was sufficient evidence that corticosteroids significantly reduce the risk of premature birth. By 1989 there was overwhelming evidence of the benefits of corticosteroids. However, it was not until 1991 that this evidence was implemented by clinicians – during which time tens of thousands of premature babies were affected by the use of ineffectual treatment. [4]

What is Competence and why is it Important?

Competence is a concept that incorporates a variety of domains including knowledge, skills and attitudes. [5] Health professionals may demonstrate overall competence in their relevant discipline via a four step process including; (i) knowledge, (ii) competence (specific to the task), (iii) performance, and (iv) action. [6] Apart from knowledge, skills and attitudes, competence also incorporates a health professional's problem solving skills (e.g. ability to critically think and apply clinical reasoning) and ability to work as a team member and communicate effectively, both in a written and verbal format. [7]

What is EBP Competence?

The amount of healthcare research and information published in peer-reviewed journal doubles every 10 to 15 years. [8] Databases such as PubMed, index the majority of these publications. In 2010 more than 20,000,000 research papers were indexed in PubMed. [9]

Regular use of these resources is identified as one marker for lifelong learning among healthcare professionals. [10] However, in order to be evidence-based practitioners, users need to have the skills to access, appraise, interpret and apply the evidence in practice. The practice of EBP consists of the following key steps;

1) Converting clinical scenarios into a structured answerable question,
2) Searching the literature to identify the best available evidence to answer the question,
3) Critically appraising the evidence for its validity and applicability
4) Applying the results of the appraisal into clinical practice, and
5) Evaluation/assessment of the EBP process. [2]

Each step of the EBP process requires a different level of knowledge and skill (i.e. competence).

1) Step 1 requires knowledge to construct a question using the PICO mnemonic (i.e. patient, intervention, comparison, outcome),
2) Step 2 requires the acquisition and application of literature searching skills across a variety of databases,
3) Step 3 requires a certain level of expertise in epidemiology and biostatistics,
4) Step 4 requires an ability to synthesize and communicate the results to relevant parties (i.e. health professionals, patients), and
5) Step 5 requires the health professional to evaluate the EBP process and assess its impact within the clinical context in which it was implemented. [11]

How do Healthcare Professionals Currently Gain Competency in EBP?

Few studies have explored how competency in EBP is represented across health disciplines. [12] A systematic review in 2009 identified three studies that explored EBP competency in medical health professionals. [12] Whilst all studies concluded that competency in at least one EBP skill increased, none were consistent in the educational approach implemented, or the EBP skill that was improved upon. [12]

Two studies assessing EBP competence in allied health professionals also differed in educational approach; with both concluding little change in EBP competence. [12] It was noteworthy that all reported educational interventions were didactic in their construction and implementation. [12]

Although traditional continuing medical education (CME) seminars adopt a didactic method of teaching, current research indicates that this does not significantly alter the behaviour of health professionals. [13, 14] Rather, a combination of strategies is required if evidence is to be successfully implemented in the healthcare system. [13, 14]

Such an implementation strategy must be tailored to suit the targeted population and issue and should adopt a variety of modalities including; traditional CME seminars, formal conferences and/or workshops, academic detailing, practice based interventions, audit with feedback and reminders. [13, 14]

These implementation strategies also need to account for non-educational variables that affect health professional behaviour. Competency in EBP is one component however, attitudes and implementation of these skills is also influenced by the characteristics of the health professional, the practice setting and patient factors. [14]

How can EBP be used in Knowledge Transfer?

Knowledge transfer aims to implement research evidence, and high quality information, to specific stakeholders using tailored interventions that account for various cultural and organizational barriers and enablers to this process. In this instance, EBP can be considered an individualized version of the knowledge transfer process. In undertaking the five steps of EBP, health professionals must identify the information gap, identify the relevant evidence, critically appraise the evidence, implement it within the clinical context and finally evaluate its effectiveness in facilitating positive change. During each of these steps, the clinician must assess the barriers and facilitators to implanting knowledge transfer and its implication on the next EBP step (Table I).

Table I. Barriers and facilitators to the EBP process in knowledge transfer

EBP process	Barriers &facilitators
Converting clinical scenarios into a structured answerable question	Understanding of how to construct a question using the PICO structure
Searching the literature to identify the best available evidence to answer the question	Skills associated with constructing a search strategy across a variety of databases
Critically appraising the evidence for its validity and applicability	Methodological understanding of quantitative research methodology
Applying the results of the appraisal into clinical practice	Understanding of individual patient, and organisational values and circumstances
Evaluation/assessment of the EBP process	Research skill in evaluating the effectiveness of the implemented EBP within the clinical scenario

A Case Scenario

Mr PT is a 65-year-old man who has painful osteoarthritis in both knees and no other major medical conditions. Although he can still carry out his activities of daily living, he has limited mobility and reports pain at rest. He has previously consuming 4 grams/day acetaminophen, which has provided minimal pain relief. The patient is eager to try a different medication. His treating clinician believes that non-steroidal anti-inflammatory drugs (NSAIDs) may be beneficial, but is wary of the gastrointestinal side effects, and wonder whether topical application of NSAIDs might be beneficial. In this case scenario the clinician would be able to complete all five EBP steps and implement the evidence in treating the patient. By completing the first three EBP steps, the clinician might find evidence from a systematic review such. [15] Critical appraisal of the evidence would indicate that it is high quality, with the results suggesting that topical NSAIDs are only effective in temporary relief of OA of the knee (1-2 weeks), with no difference in adverse events when compared to oral NSAIDs. Steps 4 of the EBP process would be to apply this evidence to the patient and identify an appropriate treatment plan. The final step would require an evaluation of the entire process. Whilst the EBP process might be somewhat consuming in the first instance, the clinician and the patient have both benefited from the knowledge that has been transferred from the research context into clinical practice. Additionally, both parties have the opportunity to further propagate their newfound information to other colleagues and peers, further facilitating the knowledge transfer process.

How Can EBP Impact Upon Patient Care?

Improving health professional competency in EBP ensures that health decision making, be it from a research, policy or clinical perspective, is translated into practice to benefit the greater population. Health professionals who are competent in EBP are able to base healthcare decisions on an informed evidence base. Such health professionals will be able to provide the best care to their patients and also reduce the burden of implementing ineffective healthcare interventions on the healthcare system. For example, the Australian government currently recommends the vaccination of older Australians and individuals aged six months and over with medical conditions predisposing to severe influenza. [16] However, current evidence-based research indicates the effectiveness of influenza vaccines for people aged 65 years or older is of poor quality and provides no guidance regarding its safety, efficacy or effectiveness. [17] Current evidence indicates that provision of the influenza vaccine to children over two years of age is beneficial; however there is a lack of evidence in children under two years of age. [18]In 2004, the non-steroidal anti-inflammatory drug (NSAID) Rofecoxib (also known generically as Vioxx), was withdrawn from sales due to research indicating an increased risk of cardiovascular risk in patients taking the drug. [19]

Critically, there was significant research evidence by 2000 that demonstrated that Rofecoxib was harmful to patients. [20]By the time it was withdrawn in 2004 an estimated 80 million people had consumed the drug. [20]These two examples illustrate how health professionals, who are competent in the skills of EBP, would be able to discriminate between effective and potentially effective healthcare interventions. Promoting the life-long learning skills via EBP, provides a de facto method of promoting knowledge transfer at the individual clinician level, thereby providing a better economic, social and health related outcomes.

CONCLUSION

Evidence based practice provides users with a skill set to continuously manage life-long learning in their selected health discipline. These same EBP skills provide users with a unique opportunity to actively engage in the knowledge transfer process. To date, no formal evaluation of this evidence based practice-knowledge transfer (EBP-KT) nexus has been conducted.

Rigorous studies are required to evaluate the effectiveness of this EBP-KT within different organizational settings and within different patient cohorts. Additionally, research is required to identify what impact, if any, the level of EBP competence (be it novice, intermediate or expert) has upon the users' ability to use their EBP skill in partaking in the knowledge transfer process.

REFERENCES

[1] Guyatt G: Evidence-Based Medicine. *ACP Journal Club* 1991, A-16:114.

[2] Sackett D, Straus S, Richardson W, Rosenberg W: *Evidence-based medicine.* Edinburgh: Churchill Livingstone; 2000.

[3] Glasziou P: Why is evidence-based medicine important?*EBM notebook* 2006, 11: 133-135.

[4] The Cochrane Collaboration: Cochrane Collaboration logo [Available at: http://www.cochrane.org/about-us/history/our-logo (Accessed 18/10/2011)].

[5] Holmboe E, Hawkins R: Methods for evaluating the clinical competence of residents in internal medicine. *Annals of Internal Medicine* 1998, 129:42-48.

[6] Miller G: The assessment of clinical skills/competence/performance. *Academic Medicine* 1990, 65:S63-67.

[7] McAllister M: Competency standards: clarifying the issues. *Contemporary Nurse* 1998, 7:131-137.

[8] Hook O: History, electronic journals and impact factors. *Scandanavian Journal of Rehabilitative Medicine* 1999, 31:3-7.

[9] US National Library of Medicine and National Institutes of Health. *Pub. Med.* [Available at: http://www.ncbi.nlm.nih.gov/pubmed/ (Accessed 18/10/2011)].

[10] Hojat M, Nasca T, Frsiby A, Veloski J, Gonnella J: An operational measure of physician lifelong learning:its development, components and preliminary psychometric data. *Medical Teacher* 2003, 25:433-437.

[11] Rosenberg W, Donald A: Evidence based medicine: an approach to clinical problem-solving. *BMJ* 1995, 310:1122-1126.

[12] Ilic D: Teaching Evidence-based Practice: Perspectives from the Undergraduate and Post-graduate Viewpoint. *Annals of Academic Medicine Singapore* 2009, 38:559-563.

[13] Grimshaw J, Eccles M: Is evidence-based implementation of evidence-based care possible?*MJA* 2004, 1810:S50-51.

[14] Davis D, O'Brien M, Freemantle N, Wolf F, Mazmanian P, Taylor-Vaisey A: Impact of formal continuing medical education: do conferences, workshops, rounds, and other traditional continuing education activities change physician behavior or health care outcomes?*JAMA* 1999, 282:867-874.

[15] Lin J, Zhang W, Doherty M: Efficacy of topical non-steroidal anti-inflammatory drugs in the treatment of osteoarthritis: meta-analysis of randomised controlled trials. *BMJ* 2004, 329:324-329.

[16] Department of Health and Ageing. *Immunise Australia Program.* Immunise Australia Program. [Available at: http://www.health.gov.au/internet/immunise/publishing.nsf/content/immunise-influenza (Accessed 18/10/2011)].

[17] Jefferson T, Di Pietrantonj C, Al-Ansary L, Ferroni E, Thorning S, Thomas R: Vaccines for preventing influenza in the elderly. *Cochrane Database of Systematic Reviews* 2010, Issue 2. Art. No.: CD004876. DOI: 10.1002/14651858.CD004876.pub3.

[18] Jefferson T, Rivetti A, Harnden A, Di Pietrantonj C, Demicheli V: Vaccines for preventing influenza in healthy children. *Cochrane Database of Systematic Reviews* 2008, Issue 2. Art. No.: CD004879. DOI: 10.1002/14651858.CD004879.pub3.

[19] Merck. Merck announces voluntary worldwide withdrawal of VIOXX®. [Available at: http://www.merck.com/newsroom/vioxx/pdf/vioxx_press_release_final.pdf (Accessed 18/10/2011)]

[20] Juni P, Nartey L, Reichenbach S, Sterchi R, Dieppe P, Egger M: Risk of cardiobascular events and rofecoxib: cumulative meta-analysis. *Lancet* 2004, 364:2021-2029.

In: Knowledge Transfer: Practices, Types and Challenges
Editor: Dragan Ilic
ISBN: 978-1-62081-538-0

Chapter 5

PARAMETRIC LINK MODELS FOR KNOWLEDGE TRANSFER IN STATISTICAL LEARNING

***F. Beninel*[1], *C. Biernacki*[2], *C. Bouveyron*[3], *J. Jacques*[*2] *and A. Lourme*[4]**
[1]CREST-ENSAI, Bruz, France
[2]UniversitÃ© Lille 1 & CNRS & INRIA, Lille, France
[3]UniversitÃ© Paris 1 PanthÃ©on-Sorbonne, Paris, France
[4]UniversitÃ© de Pau et des Pays de l'Adour, Pau, France

Abstract

When a statistical model is designed in a prediction purpose, a major assumption is the absence of evolution in the modeled phenomenon between the training and the prediction stages. Thus, training and future data must be in the same feature space and must have the same distribution. Unfortunately, this assumption turns out to be often false in real-world applications. For instance, biological motivations could lead to classify individuals from a given species when only individuals from another species are available for training. In regression, we would sometimes use a predictive model for data having not exactly the same distribution that the training data used for estimating the model. This chapter presents techniques for transfering a statistical model estimated from a *source* population to a *target* population. Three tasks of statistical learning are considered: Probabilistic classification (parametric and semi-parametric), linear regression (including mixture of regressions) and model-based clustering (Gaussian and Student). In each situation, the knowledge transfer is carried out by introducing parametric links between both populations. The use of such transfer techniques would improve the performance of learning by avoiding much expensive data labeling efforts.

Keywords: Adaptive estimation, link between populations, transfer learning, classification, regression, clustering, EM algorithm, applications AMS Subject Classification: 62H30, 62J99 on the last page

---

*E-mail address: julien.jacques@polytech-lille.fr

1. Introduction

Statistical learning [17] is a key tool for many science and application areas since it allows to explain and to predict diverse phenomena from the observation of related data. It leads to a wide variety of methods, depending on the particular problem at hand. Examples of such problems are numerous:

- Examples E_1: In *Credit Scoring*, predict the behavior of borrowers to pay back loan, on the basis of information known about these customers; In *Medicine*, predict the risk of lung cancer recurrence for a patient treated for a first cancer, on the basis of the type of treatment used for the first cancer and on clinical and demographic measurements for that patient.

- Examples E_2: In *Economics*, predict the housing price on the basis of several housing descriptive variables; In *Finance*, predict the profitability of a financial asset six months after purchase.

- Examples E_3: In *Marketing*, create customers groups according to their purchase history in order to target a marketing campaign; In *Biology*, identify groups in a sample of birds described by some biometric features which finally reveal the presence of different genders.

In a typical statistical learning problem, a response variable $y \in \mathcal{Y}$ has to be predicted from a set of d feature variables (or covariates) $\boldsymbol{x} = (x_1, \ldots, x_d) \in \mathcal{X}$. Spaces $\mathcal{X}$ and $\mathcal{Y}$ are usually quantitative or categorical. It is also possible to have heterogeneity in features variables (both quantitative and categorical for instance). The analysis always relies on a training dataset $\mathcal{S} = (\mathbf{x}, \mathbf{y})$, in which the response and feature variables are observed for a set of n individuals which are respectively denoted by $\mathbf{x} = (\boldsymbol{x}_1, \ldots, \boldsymbol{x}_n)$ and $\mathbf{y} = (y_1, \ldots, y_n)$. Using $\mathcal{S}$, a predictive model is built in order to predict the response variable for a new individual, for which the covariates $\boldsymbol{x}$ are observed but not the response y. This typical situation is called *supervised* learning. In particular, if $\mathcal{Y}$ is a categorical space, it corresponds to a *discriminant analysis* situation; It aims to solve problems which look like Examples E_1. If $\mathcal{Y}$ is a quantitative space, it corresponds to a *regression* situation and aims to solve problems similar to Examples E_2. Note also that if $\mathbf{y}$ is only partially known in $\mathcal{S}$, it exhibits what is called *semi-supervised* learning.

Another typical statistical learning problem consists in predicting the whole responses $\mathbf{y}$ while having never observe them. In this case only the feature variables are known, thus $\mathcal{S} = \mathbf{x}$, and it corresponds to an *unsupervised* learning situation. If $\mathcal{Y}$ is restricted to a categorical space (the most frequent case), it consists in a *clustering* purpose, related problems being illustrated by Examples E_3.

In this chapter, we focus on statistical modeling for solving as well supervised and unsupervised learning. Many classical probabilistic methods exist and we will give useful references, when necessary, throughout the chapter. Thus, the reader interested for such references is invited to have a look in related sections below.

A main assumption in supervised learning is the absence of evolution in the modeled phenomenon between the training of the model and the prediction of the response for a new individual. More precisely, the new individual is assumed to arise from the same statistical population than the training one. In unsupervised learning, it is also implicitly assumed that all individuals arise from the same population. Unfortunately, such classical hypotheses may not hold in many realistic situations as reflected by revisited Examples E_1 to E_3:

- Examples E_1^*: In *Credit Scoring*, the statistical scoring model has been trained on a dataset of customers but is used to predict behavior of non-customers; In *Medicine*, the risk of lung cancer recurrence is learned for an European patient but will be applied to an Asian patient.

- Examples E_2^*: In *Economics*, a real-estate agency implanted for a long time on the US East Coast aims to conquer new markets by opening several agencies on the West Coast but both markets are quite different; In *Finance*, expertise in financial asset of the past year is surely different from the current one.

- Examples E_3^*: In *Marketing*, customers to be classified correspond in fact to a pooled panel of new and older customers; In *Biology*, different subpecies of birds are pooled together and may consequently have highly different features for the same gender.

In the supervised setting, the question is "Q_1: Is it necessary to recollect new training data and to build a new statistical learning model or can the previous training data still be useful?" In the unsupervised setting, the question is "Q_2: Is it better to perform a unique clustering on the whole data set or to perform several independant clusterings on some identified subsets?".

Question Q_1 is addressed as *transfer* learning and a general overview is given in [28]. Transfer learning techniques aim to transfer the knowledge learned on a source population Ω to a target population Ω^*, in which this knowledge will be used in a prediction purpose. These techniques are divided into two important situations: The transfer of a model *does need* or *does not need* to observe some response variables in the target domain. The first case is quoted as *inductive transfer* learning whereas the second one is quoted as *transductive transfer* learning. Usually, the classification purpose as described in Examples E_1^* can be solved by either transductive or inductive transfer learning, this choice depending on the model at hand (generative or predictive models). Contrariwise, the regression purpose as described in Examples E_2^* can be only solved by inductive transfer learning since only predictive models are involved. Question Q_2 is adressed as *unsupervised transfer* learning. It corresponds to simultaneous clustering of several samples and, thus, it concerns Examples E_3^*.

A common expected advantage of all these transfer learning techniques is a real predictive benefit since knowledge learned on the source population is used in addition to the available information on the target population. However, the common challenge is to establish a "transfer function" between the source and the target populations. In this chapter, we focus on parametric statistical models. Besides being good competitors to nonparametric models in terms of prediction, these models have the advantage of being easily interpreted by practitioners. Since parametric models will be used, it will be natural to modelize the transfer function by some parametric links. Thus, in addition to a predictive benefit, the interpretability of the link parameters will give to practitioners useful information on the evolution and the differences between the source and target populations.

This chapter is organized as follows. Section 2. presents transfer learning for different discriminant analysis contexts: Gaussian model (continuous covariates), Bernoulli model (binary covariates) and logistic model (continuous or binary covariates). Section 3. considers the transfer of regression models for a quantitative response variable in two situations: Usual regression and mixture of regressions. Finally, Section 4. proposes models to cluster simultaneously a source and a target population in two situations again: Mixtures of Gaussian and Student distributions. Each section starts with a presentation of the classical statistical model before presenting the corresponding transfer techniques, and it concludes by an application on real data.

A useful notation In the following the notation "*" will refer to the target population.

2. Parametric transfer learning in discriminant analysis

Discriminant analysis is a large methodological field covering machine learning techniques dealing with data where individuals are described by the same set of d covariates or feature vector $\boldsymbol{x}$ and a response categorical variable $y \in \mathcal{Y} = \{1,\ldots,K\}$ related to K classes, where $y = k$ if the individual described by $\boldsymbol{x}$ belongs to the kth class. In a statistical setting, the couple $(\boldsymbol{x}, y)$ is assumed to be a realization of a random vector $(\boldsymbol{X}, Y)$ where $\boldsymbol{X} = (X_1,\ldots,X_d)$. Then the n-sample $\mathcal{S} = (\mathbf{x},\mathbf{y})$ is assumed to be n i.i.d. realizations of $(\boldsymbol{X}, Y)$.

The purpose of discriminant analysis is to predict the group membership y, only on the basis of the covariates $\boldsymbol{x}$. The discriminant analysis proceeds as follows: Using $\mathcal{S}$, an allocation rule is built in order to classify non-labeled individuals. Many books explain in detail the numerous techniques related to discriminant analysis [16,17,25,29], among which the main are parametric ones, semi-parametric ones, non-parametric ones and borderline-based ones. In this section, we are interested only by parametric (Gaussian and Bernoulli distributions) and semi-parametric (logistic regression) methods.

2.1. Gaussian discriminant analysis

2.1.1. The statistical model

Gaussian discriminant analysis assumes that, conditionally to the group y, the feature variables $\boldsymbol{x} \in \mathcal{X} = \mathbb{R}^d$ arise from a random vector $\boldsymbol{X}$ distributed according to a d-variate Gaussian distribution

$$\boldsymbol{X}_{|}Y = k \sim \mathcal{N}_d(\boldsymbol{\mu}_k, \boldsymbol{\Sigma}_k),$$

where $\boldsymbol{\mu}_k \in \mathbb{R}^d$ and $\boldsymbol{\Sigma}_k \in \mathbb{R}^{d\times d}$ are respectively the associated mean and covariance matrix. The probability density of $\boldsymbol{X}$ conditionally to $Y = k$ is

$$f_k(\bullet;\boldsymbol{\mu}_k,\boldsymbol{\Sigma}_k) = \frac{1}{(2\pi)^{d/2}|\boldsymbol{\Sigma}_k|^{1/2}} \exp\left(-\frac{1}{2}(\bullet-\boldsymbol{\mu}_k)'\boldsymbol{\Sigma}_k^{-1}(\bullet-\boldsymbol{\mu}_k)\right).$$

The marginal distribution of $\boldsymbol{X}$ is then a mixture of Gaussian distributions

$$\boldsymbol{X} \sim f(\bullet;\boldsymbol{\theta}) = \sum_{k=1}^{K} \pi_k f_k(\bullet;\boldsymbol{\mu}_k,\boldsymbol{\Sigma}_k),$$

where $(\pi_1,\ldots,\pi_K)$ are the mixing proportions ($\pi_k > 0$ and $\sum_{k=1}^K \pi_k = 1$) and $\boldsymbol{\theta} = \{(\pi_k, \boldsymbol{\mu}_k, \boldsymbol{\Sigma}_k) : k = 1,\ldots,K\}$ is the whole parameter. When the costs of bad classification are assumed to be symmetric, the *Maximum A Posteriori* (MAP) rule consists in assigning a new individual $\boldsymbol{x}$ to the group $\hat{y}$ maximizing the membership conditional probability $t_{\hat{y}}(\boldsymbol{x};\boldsymbol{\theta})$:

$$\hat{y} = \underset{k\in\{1,\ldots,K\}}{\text{argmax}}\ t_k(\boldsymbol{x};\boldsymbol{\theta}), \tag{1}$$

where

$$t_k(\boldsymbol{x};\boldsymbol{\theta}) = P(Y = k|\boldsymbol{X} = \boldsymbol{x};\boldsymbol{\theta}) = \frac{\pi_k f_k(\boldsymbol{x};\boldsymbol{\alpha}_k)}{f(\boldsymbol{x};\boldsymbol{\theta})}. \tag{2}$$

In the general heteroscedastic situation (quadratic discriminant analysis or QDA), $\boldsymbol{\theta}$ is estimated by its classical empirical estimates:

$$\hat{\pi}_k = \frac{n_k}{n}, \quad \hat{\boldsymbol{\mu}}_k = \frac{1}{n_k}\sum_{\{i:y_i=k\}} \boldsymbol{x}_i, \quad \hat{\boldsymbol{\Sigma}}_k = \frac{1}{n_k - 1}\sum_{\{i:y_i=k\}} (\boldsymbol{x}_i - \hat{\boldsymbol{\mu}}_k)(\boldsymbol{x}_i - \hat{\boldsymbol{\mu}}_k)',$$

where $n_k = \text{card}\{i : y_i = k\}$ is the number of individuals of the training sample $\mathcal{S}$ belonging to the group k. In the restricted homoscedastic situation $\boldsymbol{\Sigma}_k = \boldsymbol{\Sigma}$ for all k (linear discriminant analysis or LDA), the covariance matrix is estimated by

$$\hat{\boldsymbol{\Sigma}} = \frac{1}{n-K}\sum_{k=1}^{K}\sum_{\{i:y_i=k\}} (\boldsymbol{x}_i - \hat{\boldsymbol{\mu}}_k)(\boldsymbol{x}_i - \hat{\boldsymbol{\mu}}_k)'.$$

2.1.2. The transfer learning and its estimation

Now we assume that the data consist of two samples: A first labeled n-sample $\mathcal{S} = (\mathbf{x}, \mathbf{y})$, drawn from a source population Ω, and a second unlabeled n^*-sample $\mathcal{S}^* = \mathbf{x}^*$, drawn from a target population Ω^*. Our goal is to build a classification rule for the target population using both samples $\mathcal{S}$ and $\mathcal{S}^*$. An extension to a partially-labeled target sample $\mathcal{S}^*$ will be also presented later. The source labeled sample $\mathcal{S}$ is composed by n pairs $(\boldsymbol{x}_i, y_i)$, assumed to be i.i.d. realizations of the random couple $(\boldsymbol{X}, Y)$ of distribution

$$\boldsymbol{X}_{|Y=k} \sim \mathcal{N}_d(\boldsymbol{\mu}_k, \boldsymbol{\Sigma}_k) \qquad \text{and} \qquad Y \sim \mathcal{M}_1(\pi_1,\ldots,\pi_K),$$

where $\mathcal{M}_1$ is the one-order multinomial distribution. The target unlabeled sample $\mathcal{S}^*$ is composed by n^* pairs $\boldsymbol{x}_i^*$ i.i.d. realizations of $\boldsymbol{X}^*$ with the following Gaussian mixture distribution

$$\boldsymbol{X}^* \sim f(\bullet;\boldsymbol{\theta}^*).$$

In order to use both samples $\mathcal{S}$ and $\mathcal{S}^*$ for the classification of $\mathcal{S}^*$ sample (or of any new individual $\boldsymbol{x}$ from Ω^*), the approach developped in [3] consists in establishing a stochastic relationship $\phi_k(\mathbb{R}^d \mapsto \mathbb{R}^d)$ between feature vectors of both populations conditionally to groups, *i.e.*

$$\boldsymbol{X}^*_{|Y^*=k} \overset{\mathcal{D}}{=} \phi_k(\boldsymbol{X}_{|Y=k}) = [\phi_k^1(\boldsymbol{X}_{|Y=k}),\ldots,\phi_k^d(\boldsymbol{X}_{|Y=k})],$$

where $\mathcal{D}$ means that the equality is in distribution, and ϕ_k^j, $j = 1,\ldots,d$, is an application $(\mathbb{R}^d \mapsto \mathbb{R})$. Two natural assumptions are considered:

- $\mathcal{A}_1$: The jth component $\phi_k^j(\boldsymbol{X}_{|Y=k})$ only depends on the jth component of $\boldsymbol{X}_{|Y=k}$,
- $\mathcal{A}_2$: Each ϕ_k^j is $\mathcal{C}^1$ (continuously differentiable).

As a consequence of the previous assumptions [10] derive the K relations

$$\boldsymbol{X}^*_{|Y^*=k} \stackrel{\mathcal{D}}{=} \mathbf{D}_k \boldsymbol{X}_{|Y=k} + \mathbf{b}_k \qquad (k = 1, \ldots, K) \tag{3}$$

with $\mathbf{D}_k$ a $d \times d$ real diagonal matrix and $\mathbf{b}_k$ a d dimensional real vector. Therefore, we establish the following relations between parameters of the Gaussian distributions related to populations Ω and Ω^*:

$$\boldsymbol{\mu}_k^* = \mathbf{D}_k \boldsymbol{\mu}_k + \mathbf{b}_k \qquad \text{and} \qquad \boldsymbol{\Sigma}_k^* = \mathbf{D}_k \boldsymbol{\Sigma}_k \mathbf{D}_k. \tag{4}$$

Such relations allow to determine the allocation rules for population Ω^* using parameters of feature vector distribution for individuals of Ω. Indeed, if the K pairs $(\mathbf{D}_k, \mathbf{b}_k)$ are known it is easy to derive pairs $(\boldsymbol{\mu}_k^*, \boldsymbol{\Sigma}_k^*)$ from $(\boldsymbol{\mu}_k, \boldsymbol{\Sigma}_k)$ by plug-in. In what follows we discuss issues where the pairs $(\mathbf{D}_k, \mathbf{b}_k)$ are unkwown and we propose several scenarios for estimating them.

Constrained models For identifiability reasons we impose that $\mathbf{b}_k = \mathbf{0}$ for all $k = 1, \ldots, K$. This assumption is discussed in the seminal article on transfer learning in Gaussian discriminant analysis [3], and validated on the biological application analysed in this article. The case without constraints on $\mathbf{b}_k$ is treated in [22] which provides specific computation approach for avoiding identifiability problems (see also Section 4. of the present chapter).

In order to define parsimonious and meaningful models, constraints are now imposed on the parameters of transfer $\mathbf{D}_k$ $(k = 1, \ldots, K)$:

- Model M_1: $\mathbf{D}_k = \mathbf{I}_d$: The K distributions are the same ($\mathbf{I}_d$: identity matrix of $\mathbb{R}^{d \times d}$).
- Model M_2: $\mathbf{D}_k = \alpha \mathbf{I}_d$: Transformations are feature and group independent.
- Model M_3: $\mathbf{D}_k = \mathbf{D}$: Transformations are only group independent.
- Model M_4: $\mathbf{D}_k = \alpha_k \mathbf{I}_d$: Transformations are only feature independent.
- Model M_5: $\mathbf{D}_k$ is unconstrained, *i.e.* it is the most general situation.

Model M_1 consists in using allocation rules on Ω^* based only on $\mathcal{S}$, *i.e.* we deal here with classical discriminant analysis. Models M_2 and M_3 preserve homoscedasticity and consequently an eventual linearity of the rule: If $\boldsymbol{\Sigma}_1 = \ldots = \boldsymbol{\Sigma}_K$ for Ω, then $\boldsymbol{\Sigma}_1^* = \ldots = \boldsymbol{\Sigma}_K^*$ for Ω^*. Last models M_4 and M_5 may transform linear allocation rules into quadratic ones on Ω^* with few parameters to estimate.

For each model, an additional assumption on the mixing proportions is done: They are the same in both populations or they have to be estimated in the target population. Corresponding models are quoted by M_j and respectively πM_j $(1 \leq j \leq 5)$. The number of free parameters for each model are given in Table 1.

Table 1. Number of estimated parameters for each model.

M_1	M_2	M_3	M_4	M_5	πM_1	πM_2	πM_3	πM_4	πM_5
0	1	d	K	dK	$K-1$	K	$d+K-1$	$2K-1$	$dK+K-1$

Parameter estimation A sequential *plug-in* procedure is used to estimate matrices $\mathbf{D}_1,\ldots,\mathbf{D}_K$ (and eventually $\pi_1^*,\ldots,\pi_K^*$). The corresponding estimators will depend on parameter $\boldsymbol{\theta}$ of population Ω. When this last is unknown, it is simply replaced by its estimate. Estimating all π_k^* and all $\mathbf{D}_k$ is performed by maximizing the following likelihood, under the constraints given in (4) and under the constraint of one of the previous parsimonious models M_j or πM_j $(j=1,\ldots,5)$,

$$L(\boldsymbol{\theta}^*) = \prod_{i=1}^{n^*} f(\boldsymbol{x}_i^*;\boldsymbol{\theta}^*). \tag{5}$$

A usual way to maximize the likelihood when the group membership y_i^* is unknown is to use an EM algorithm [11] which consists in iterating the two following steps:

- **E step**: Estimation of the group membership y_i^* by its expectation conditional to the observed data:

$$\hat{y}_i^* = \underset{k\in\{1,\ldots,K\}}{\operatorname{argmax}}\ t_k(\boldsymbol{x}_i^*;\boldsymbol{\mu}_k^*,\boldsymbol{\Sigma}_k^*).$$

- **M step**: Computation of the parameter $\boldsymbol{\theta}^*$ maximizing, under the constraints given in (4) and under the constraint of a given parsimonious models (M_j or πM_j), the following completed log-likelihood:

$$\ell_c(\boldsymbol{\theta}^*) = \sum_{k=1}^{K}\sum_{\{i:y_i^*=k\}} \ln\left[\pi_k^* f_k(\boldsymbol{x}_i^*;\boldsymbol{\alpha}_k^*)\right].$$

The EM algorithm stops when the growth of the likelihood is lower than a fixed threshold.

In order to choose between several constrained models, the BIC criterion (*Bayesian Information Criterion*, [31]) is used:

$$\text{BIC} = -2\ln\ell + |\boldsymbol{\theta}^*|\ln n^* \tag{6}$$

where ℓ is the maximum log-likelihood value and $|\boldsymbol{\theta}^*|$ denotes the number of continuous model parameters in $\boldsymbol{\theta}^*$ (see Table 1). The model leading to the minimum BIC value is retained. Note that the BIC criterion is faster to compute that any cross-validation criterion.

2.1.3. A biological application

Data Data are related to seabirds from Cory's Shearwater *Calanectris diomedea* species breeding in the Mediterranean and North Atlantic, where presumably contrasted oceanographic conditions have led to the existence of marked subspecies differing in size as well as coloration and behavior [32]. Subspecies are *borealis*, living in the Atlantic islands (the Azores, Canaries, *etc.*), *diomedea*, living in the Mediterranean islands (Balearics, Corsica, *etc.*), and *edwardsii*, from the Cape Verde Islands.

A sample of *borealis* ($n = 206$, 45% females) was measured using skins in several National Museums. Five morphological variables are measured: Culmen (bill length), tarsus, wing and tail lengths, and culmen depth. Similarly, a sample of subspecies *diomedea* ($n = 38$, 58% females) was measured using the same set of variables. Figure 1 plots culmen depth and tarsus length for *borealis* and *diomedea* samples.

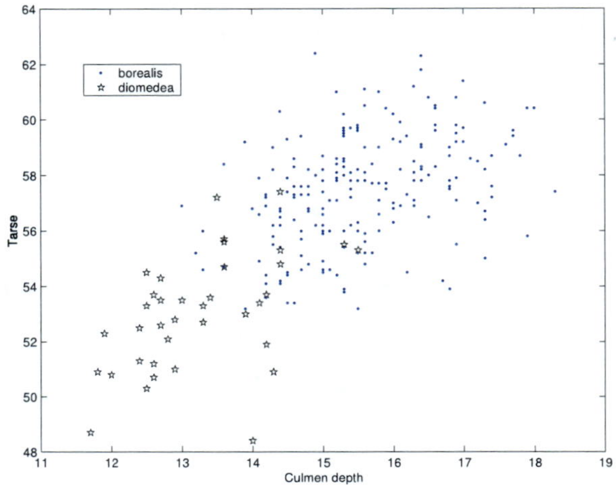

Figure 1. *Borealis* and *diomedea* for variables culmen depth and tarsus length.

In the following, we consider the *borealis* sample as being the source labeled population, and the *diomedea* as being the target population (non-labeled or partially-labeled). In reality, in our data, both samples are sexed but sex of *diomedea* will be only used to measure quality of results provided by the proposed method.

Results in the non-sexed case We consider in this section that all *diomedea* specimen are non-sexed. Linear discriminant analysis model is selected for the *borealis* population. We apply parameters estimated by the *borealis* sample using the 10 models to the non-sexed *diomedea* sample. Results, empirical error rate (deduced from the true partition of *diomedea*) and BIC value, are given for each model in Table 2. Moreover, empirical error rate of the cluster analysis situation is reported at the last column of Table 2. The clustering procedure (see for instance [9]) consists in estimating the Gaussian mixture parameters of the non-sexed sample *diomedea* without using the *borealis* sample.
High error rates are generally obtained with standard discriminant analysis (models M_1 and πM_1) and with standard cluster analysis, as compared to the other transfer learning models. The best model selected by the empirical error rate is πM_3. This model preserves homoscedasticity, a relevant property since both discriminant rules selected by cross-validation criterion separately on each sample $\mathcal{S}$ and $\mathcal{S}^*$ (not reported here) were homoscedastic (LDA). Moreover it indicates that the proportion of females is not the same in the two samples. Model selected by the BIC criterion is M_3 and the error rate is the second best value. So, transformation from *borealis* to *diomedea* seems to be sex-independent but

Table 2. Empirical error rate (error) and BIC value (BIC) in the non-sexed case

model	M_1	M_2	M_3	M_4	M_5
error	42.11	31.58	18.43	28.95	21.06
BIC	-753.49	-502.13	**-451.51**	-503.74	-457.69

model	πM_1	πM_2	πM_3	πM_4	πM_5	clustering
error	42.11	42.11	**15.79**	42.11	21.06	44.73
BIC	-725.24	-489.43	-453.20	-491.23	-459.51	–

not variable-independent. It should be noted also that BIC's value for πM_3 is very close to the one for M_3.

Results in the partially-sexed case We consider in this section that two labels (therefore 5.26% of the data set) are known in the *diomedea* sample, thus a part $\tilde{\mathbf{y}}^*$ of $\mathbf{y}^*$ is known and $\mathcal{S}^* = (\mathbf{x}^*, \tilde{\mathbf{y}}^*)$. Empirical error rate is obtained for the 36 *a priori* non-sexed birds. The two labels are choosen at random 30 times and, so, it leads to 30 partially-sexed samples. The 10 models and cluster analysis (using also this new sex information, what leads to a semi-supervised situation) are applied successively to the 30 partially-sexed *diomedea* samples. Mean of the error rate and of the BIC criterion are displayed in Table 3.

Table 3. Mean on the 30 samples of the empirical error rate (error) and the BIC value (BIC) in the partially-sexed case

model	M_1	M_2	M_3	M_4	M_5
error	42.41	31.94	18.70	29.91	18.98
BIC	-753.49	-502.13	**-451.56**	-503.92	-457.95

model	πM_1	πM_2	πM_3	πM_4	πM_5	clustering
error	42.41	42.69	**15.37**	42.69	20.93	21.13
BIC	-725.99	-489.95	-453.32	-491.77	-460.74	–

Partial information on sex provides lower error rates in models πM_3, πM_5, M_5 and the clustering method, with the model πM_3 still being the best. The BIC criterion still selects the model M_3 (with a low error rate) and then πM_3. We note that, except model M_5, only adapted models improve thanks to this new label knowledge. Moreover, the more complex the model is, the more the error of classification strongly decreases. This is the case for clustering: It has a good improvement in this example, coming from the last rank to a level close to πM_5.

2.2. Discriminant analysis for binary data

2.2.1. The statistical model

We now consider discriminant analysis for binary feature variables, so $\mathcal{X} = \{0,1\}^d$. If the Gaussian assumption is common for quantitative feature variables, binary feature x_j is commonly assumed to arise from a random variable X_j having, conditionally on Y, a Bernoulli distribution $\mathcal{B}(\alpha_{kj})$ of parameter α_{kj} $(0 < \alpha_{kj} < 1)$:

$$X_{j|Y=k} \sim \mathcal{B}(\alpha_{kj}) \quad (j = 1,\dots,d). \tag{7}$$

Using the assumption of conditional independence of the explanatory variables [8, 13], the probability density function of $\boldsymbol{X}$, conditionally on Y, is:

$$f_k(\boldsymbol{x};\boldsymbol{\alpha}_k) = \prod_{j=1}^{d} \alpha_{kj}^{x_j}(1-\alpha_{kj})^{1-x_j}, \tag{8}$$

where $\boldsymbol{\alpha}_k = (\alpha_{k1},\dots,\alpha_{kd})$. The mixing proportions π_k and the whole parameter $\boldsymbol{\theta} = \{(\pi_k,\boldsymbol{\alpha}_k), k = 1,\dots,K\}$ are then defined similarly to the previous Gaussian situation. Maximum likelihood (ML) estimates of all α_{kj} are simply given by the following relative empirical frequencies:

$$\hat{\alpha}_{kj} = \frac{\text{card}\{i : y_i = k, x_{ij} = 1\}}{n_k}.$$

The estimation of any y is then obtain by the MAP principle given in (1), $\boldsymbol{\theta}$ being plug-in by its estimate (estimate of the mixing proportion π_k are the same as in the Gaussian situation).

2.2.2. The transfer learning

Defining a transfer function Feature variables in the target population Ω^* are assumed to have the same distribution as (7) but with possibly different parameters α^*_{kj}

$$X^*_{j|Y^*=k} \sim \mathcal{B}(\alpha^*_{kj}).$$

In a multinormal context, the transfer learning challenge has been reached by considering a linear stochastic relationship between the source Ω and the target Ω^*. This link was not only justified (under very few assumptions) but also intuitive [3]. In the binary context, such an intuitive relationship seems more difficult to exhibit. The idea developed in [21] is to assume that the binary variables result from the discretization of some latent Gaussian variables. From a stochastic link between the latent variables analogous to (3), the following link between the parameters α^*_{kj} of Ω^* and α_{kj} of Ω is obtained:

$$\alpha^*_{kj} = \Phi\Big(\delta_{kj}\,\Phi^{-1}(\alpha_{kj}) + \lambda_j\gamma_{kj}\Big), \tag{9}$$

where Φ is the cumulative density function of $\mathcal{N}(0,1)$, $\delta_{kj} \in \mathbb{R}^+ \setminus \{0\}$, $\lambda_j \in \{-1,1\}$ and $\gamma_{kj} \in \mathbb{R}$. Note that this relationship corresponds to a linear link between the *probit* functions of both α_{kj} and α^*_{kj}.

Conditionally to the fact that α_{kj} are known (they will be estimated in practice), estimation of the Kd continuous parameters α^*_{kj} is thus obtained from estimates of the link parameters δ_{kj}, γ_{kj} and λ_j between Ω and Ω^* (plug-in method). However, estimating the number of parameters for the link map is $2Kd$ and one thus obtains that the model is overparameterized. This fact should not be surprising since the underlying Gaussian model is by far more complex (in terms of the number of parameters) than the Bernoulli model. Hence there is a need to reduce the number of free continuous parameters in (9), and [21] propose constrained models imposing natural additional constraints on the transformation between both populations Ω and Ω^*.

Constrained models The parameters δ_{kj} ($1 \leq k \leq K$ and $1 \leq j \leq d$) will be successively constrained to be equal to 1 (denoted by 1), to be class- and dimension-independent (δ), to be only class-dependent (δ_k) or only dimension-dependent (δ_j). In the same way, γ_{kj} can be constrained to be equal to 0, γ (constant w.r.t. k and j), γ_k (constant w.r.t. j) or γ_j (constant w.r.t. k). Thus, 16 models can be defined and indexed using the *ad hoc* notation summarized in Table 4. For these 16 models, as for the Gaussian case, the assumption on

Table 4. Constrained models for binary discriminant analysis transfer learning

	0	γ	γ_j	γ_k
1	$1\,0$	1γ	$1\gamma_j$	$1\gamma_k$
δ	$1\,0$	$\delta\gamma$	$\delta\gamma_j$	$\delta\gamma_k$
δ_j	$\delta_j 0$	$\delta_j\gamma$	$\delta_j\gamma_j$	$\delta_j\gamma_k$
δ_k	$\delta_k 0$	$\delta_k\gamma$	$\delta_k\gamma_j$	$\delta_k\gamma_k$

the group proportions is also taken into account: For instance, an equal proportion model is quoted $\delta_k\gamma_k$ and a free proportion model is quoted $\pi\delta_k\gamma_k$. The number of constrained models is thus growing to 32. The ML estimation of the parameter $\boldsymbol{\theta}^*$ is carried out by the EM algorithm under the link constraint (9) and also w.r.t. the considered model on the link parameters. Then, the choice between these 32 models can be performed by the BIC criterion given in (6).

2.2.3. Biological application

In this application birds from the species *puffins* are considered, and the goal is to predict their sex [7]. Two groups of subspecies are considered: The first one is composed of subspecies living in Pacific Islands – *subalaris* (Galapagos Island), *polynesial*, *dichrous* (Enderbury and Palau Islands) and *gunax* – and the second one is composed of subspecies living in Atlantic Islands – *boydi* (Cap Verde Islands). Here, the difference between populations is the geographical range (Pacific *vs.* Atlantic Islands). A sample of Pacific birds ($n = 171$) was measured using skins in several National Museums. Four variables are measured on these birds: Coller, stripe and piping (absence or presence for these three variables) and under-caudal (self couloured or not). Similarly, a sample of Atlantic birds ($n = 19$) was measured using the same set of variables. Like in the previous example, two groups are present (males and females) and the sex of all the birds is known.

Pacific birds are chosen as the source population and Atlantic ones as the target population. Choosing Atlantic birds as the target population corresponds to a realistic situation because it could be hazardous to perform a clustering process on a sample of such a small size. This is a typical situation where the proposed methodology could be expected to provide a parsimonious and meaningful alternative. According to the biologist who provided the data, the morphological variables which are used in this application are not very discriminative, and then one can not expect that the error rate will be better than $40-45\%$.

The 32 transfer learnings models for binary discrimination, among which standard discriminant analysis $1\,0$, are applied on these data and the results are presented in Table 5. Clustering is also applied, and the obtained error rate is 49.05%. The best transfer learning

Table 5. Classification error rates (%) and value of the BIC criterion for target population of Atlantic birds with source on Pacific birds population

model	$1\,0$	1γ	$1\gamma_k$	$1\gamma_j$	$\delta 0$	$\delta\gamma$	$\delta\gamma_k$	$\delta\gamma_j$
error	50.94	**43.39**	45.28	43.39	50.94	**43.39**	45.28	45.28
BIC	212	**209**	216	224	212	**209**	216	224
model	$\delta_k 0$	$\delta_k\gamma$	$\delta_k\gamma_k$	$\delta_k\gamma_j$	$\delta_j 0$	$\delta_j\gamma$	$\delta_j\gamma_k$	$\delta_j\gamma_j$
error	45.28	45.28	52.83	45.28	45.28	52.83	50.94	50.94
BIC	210	210	215	226	225	224	227	239
model	$\pi 1 0$	$\pi 1\gamma$	$\pi 1\gamma_k$	$\pi 1\gamma_j$	$\pi\delta 0$	$\pi\delta\gamma$	$\pi\delta\gamma_k$	$\pi\delta\gamma_j$
error	45.28	50.94	50.94	45.28	45.28	50.94	50.94	45.28
BIC	213	213	220	228	213	213	220	228
model	$\pi\delta_k 0$	$\pi\delta_k\gamma$	$\pi\delta_k\gamma_k$	$\pi\delta_k\gamma_j$	$\pi\delta_j 0$	$\pi\delta_j\gamma$	$\pi\delta_j\gamma_k$	$\pi\delta_j\gamma_j$
error	45.28	45.28	47.16	45.28	45.28	52.83	45.28	52.83
BIC	214	213	213	229	228	227	224	243

model gives an error rate lower than standard discriminant analysis (50.94%) or clustering (49.05%) to classify birds according to their sex. Moreover the BIC criterion leads to choose the model with the smallest error rate. The relatively poor classification results (the minimal error rate is 43%) confirms the assumption of the biologist.

2.3. Logistic regression

2.3.1. The statistical model

Contrary to both previous approaches, logistic regression (see for instance [19, 26]) can be viewed as a partially parametric method since it models only the ratio $f_k(\boldsymbol{x})/f_{k'}(\boldsymbol{x})$ $(k \neq k')$ instead of modeling each single group distribution $f_k(\boldsymbol{x})$. Here, we study the case where covariates $\boldsymbol{x}$ include d components which are continuous and/or binary. The general categorical case (more than two levels for some components of $\boldsymbol{x}$) is easily taken into account by replacing each $r \geq 2$ levels covariate by $r-1$ binary covariates. We consider also that K groups have to be discriminated. Following the conventional but arbitrary choice of the Kth group as a base group, the logistic model fundamentally assumes that

$$\ln \frac{f_k(\boldsymbol{x})}{f_K(\boldsymbol{x})} = \beta^0_{0k} + \boldsymbol{\beta}'_k \boldsymbol{x}$$

where $\beta_{0k}^0 \in \mathbb{R}$ and $\boldsymbol{\beta}_k = (\beta_{1k}, \ldots, \beta_{dk})' \in \mathbb{R}^d$ $(k = 1, \ldots, K-1)$. Equivalently, it can be written by using the conditional membership probabilities $t_k(\boldsymbol{x}; \boldsymbol{\beta})$

$$\ln \frac{t_k(\boldsymbol{x}; \boldsymbol{\beta})}{t_K(\boldsymbol{x}; \boldsymbol{\beta})} = \beta_{0k} + \boldsymbol{\beta}_k' \boldsymbol{x}$$

where $\beta_{0k} = \beta_{0k}^0 + \ln(\pi_k / \pi_K)$ and $\boldsymbol{\beta} = (\beta_{01}, \ldots, \beta_{0K-1}, \boldsymbol{\beta}_1, \ldots, \boldsymbol{\beta}_{K-1})'$. It leads to the following "logistic-like" expression of conditional membership probabilities

$$t_k(\boldsymbol{x}; \boldsymbol{\beta}) = \frac{\exp(\beta_{0k} + \boldsymbol{\beta}_k' \boldsymbol{x})}{1 + \sum_{h=1}^{K-1} \exp(\beta_{0h} + \boldsymbol{\beta}_h' \boldsymbol{x})}.$$

This expression highlights the predictive focus of this model: Only useful terms for predicting the group membership (the $t_k(\boldsymbol{x}; \boldsymbol{\beta})$'s) are modeled whatever be the way the covariates $\boldsymbol{x}$ are generated. In particular, the logistic assumption includes a wide variety of families of distributions: Multivariate homoscedastic normal distributions, multivariate discrete distributions following the log-linear model with equal interaction terms, joint distributions of continuous and discrete variables of both but not necessarily independent, truncated versions of them. It implies some high flexibility which is highly appreciated by lots of practitioners in many different fields such Credit Scoring, Medicine, *etc.*

The whole parameter $\boldsymbol{\beta}$ has to be estimated from a n sample $\mathcal{S} = (\mathbf{x}, \mathbf{y})$. As previously noticed, covariates $\mathbf{x}$ arise from an unspecified mixture distribution of K groups. Then, conditionally to $\boldsymbol{x}_i$, each y_i is independently drawn from a random vector Y following the K-modal conditional multinomial distribution of order one

$$Y_{|\mathbf{X} = \boldsymbol{x}} \sim \mathcal{M}_1(t_1(\boldsymbol{x}; \boldsymbol{\beta}), \ldots, t_K(\boldsymbol{x}; \boldsymbol{\beta})).$$

With this sampling scheme, the (conditional) log-likelihood to be maximized is given by

$$\ell(\boldsymbol{\beta}) = \sum_{k=1}^{K} \sum_{\{i : y_i = k\}} \ln t_k(\boldsymbol{x}_i; \boldsymbol{\beta}).$$

No closed-formed solution exists but the log-likelihood being globally concave it can have at most one maximum. A numerical optimization algorithm has to be used and generally a Newton-Raphson procedure is retained with starting parameter $\boldsymbol{\beta} = \mathbf{0}$. Note that the ML estimates do not exist when complete or quasi-complete separation occurs.

2.3.2. Transfer learning and its estimation

In case where the sample size is small, the ML estimates of the model parameters may be of poor accuracy. It may not even exist since complete or quasi-complete separation is expected to be more frequent for small sample size. In such situations, two standard solutions occur: Either some restrictions have to be made on the model by constraining the model parameters, or the sample size has to be increased what may be difficult in many real situations (unavailable or too expensive new labeled data). An original intermediate solution is to transfer some information from another logistic regression model, estimated on a source population for which the available data are more numerous, to the previous logistic regression model. Let be Ω the source population with associated sample $\mathcal{S} = (\mathbf{x}, \mathbf{y})$ and parameter $\boldsymbol{\beta}$. Let be Ω^* the target population with associated sample $\mathcal{S}^* = (\mathbf{x}^*, \mathbf{y}^*)$ and parameter $\boldsymbol{\beta}^*$. Note that, in this regression case, all $\mathbf{y}^*$ have to be known since some $\boldsymbol{x}^*$ without its corresponding y^* value is useless in such predictive models.

Three questions naturally arise from this general idea (in italic font) with the proposed associated answers (in normal font):

1. *Why both populations Ω and Ω^* are not unrelated?* A good indicator of possible relationship between both populations is that (i) covariates $\boldsymbol{x}$ and $\boldsymbol{x}^*$ are equal or at least of same meaning and (ii) response variables y and y^* are equal or at least of same meaning.

2. *Which information is already available on $\boldsymbol{\beta}$?* An accurate estimate $\hat{\boldsymbol{\beta}}$ on $\boldsymbol{\beta}$ is easily available, typically from a sample $\mathcal{S}$ of size n greater than n^*.

3. *How both parameters $\boldsymbol{\beta}$ and $\boldsymbol{\beta}^*$ are linked?* A collection of simple, realistic, parsimonious and meaningful parametric links $\{\phi\}$ between both model parameters has to be proposed:

$$\boldsymbol{\beta}^* = \phi(\boldsymbol{\beta}).$$

One of the simplest link ϕ is affine. At this step it is fundamental to remind that $\boldsymbol{\beta}$ includes two kinds of parameters: The intercept parameters β_{0k} which have a translation effect on covariates $\boldsymbol{x}$ and the scale parameters $\boldsymbol{\beta}_k$ which have a scaling effect on covariates $\boldsymbol{x}$ ($k = 1, \ldots, K-1$). Thus it is meaningful to constraint the affine link ϕ to model a translation between β_{0k} and β^*_{0k} and to model a scaling between $\boldsymbol{\beta}_k$ and $\boldsymbol{\beta}_k{}^*$. Such a mapping is written

$$\beta^*_{0k} = \beta_{0k} + \delta_k \quad \text{and} \quad \boldsymbol{\beta}^*_k = \Lambda_k \boldsymbol{\beta}_k$$

where $\delta_k \in \mathbb{R}$ and Λ_k is a $d \times d$ diagonal matrix. Obviously, this model corresponds only to a reparameterization of the initial *logistic parameter* $\boldsymbol{\beta}$ into a *link parameter* (δ_k, Λ_k) ($k = 1, \ldots, K-1$). However, it is now possible to propose some meaningful and parsimonious restrictions on this link. In this aim, we propose the following constraints on (δ_k, Λ_k) inspired by the work of [2]:

- Three constraints on the translation δ_k:
  - $\delta_k = 0$: Both logistic models share a common intercept (simplest case);
  - $\delta_k = \delta$: Translation between both regressions is group independent;
  - δ_k free: Translation between both regressions is free (most general case).
- Five constraints on the scaling Λ_k:
  - $\Lambda_k = I$: Both logistic models share a common scaling (simplest case);
  - $\Lambda_k = \lambda I$: Scaling between both regressions is covariate and group independent;
  - $\Lambda_k = \lambda_k I$: Scaling between both regressions is covariate independent;
  - $\Lambda_k = \Lambda I$: Scaling between both regressions is group independent;

- Λ_k free: Scaling between both regressions is free (most general case).

All the previous constraints on δ_k and Λ_k can be combined and it leads to 15 models of constraints on the whole link parameter (δ_k, Λ_k). These models are noted $0I$, $\delta\lambda I$, $\delta_k\Lambda_k$,... Table 6 displays the number of parameters for each of them.

Table 6. Number of free parameters for each of the 15 models linking two logistic models

Number of parameters		Λ_k				
		I	λI	$\lambda_k I$	Λ	Λ_k
δ_k	0	0	1	$K-1$	d	$d(K-1)$
	δ	1	2	K	$d+1$	$d(K-1)+1$
	δ_k	$K-1$	K	$2(K-1)$	$K+d-1$	$(d+1)(K-1)$

We can notice some particular models:

- The simplest model $0I$ corresponds to set $\boldsymbol{\beta} = \boldsymbol{\beta}^*$;
- The most compex model $\delta_k\Lambda_k$ corresponds to unlinked parameters $\boldsymbol{\beta}$ and $\boldsymbol{\beta}^*$;
- If $K = 2$, models indexed by k are equivalent to group independent models, so only 6 different models exist in this case: $0I$, $0\lambda I$, 0Λ, δI, $\delta\lambda I$, $\delta\Lambda$;
- If $d = 1$, models including $\Lambda_{(k)}$ are equivalent to models including $\lambda_{(k)}$, so only 9 different models exist in this case.

Conditionally to $\boldsymbol{\beta}$, estimating $\boldsymbol{\beta}^*$ for a given model is easy. Indeed, since the traditional log-likelihood $\ell(\boldsymbol{\beta}^*)$ is concave and since all models correspond to linear constraints on $\boldsymbol{\beta}^*$, the resulting log-likelihood function to be maximized is also concave. As a consequence, there exists again at most one maximum and any optimisation algorithm subject to linear constraint can be involved.

Selecting a model can be performed either by some standard cross-validation methods or by using the BIC criterion [31].

2.3.3. Biological and Marketing applications

The last question that has to be raised about the proposed models is "are the link models realistic?" Applications are now useful for assessing this essential property. All applications will share the same following design experiment process:

1. $\boldsymbol{\beta}$ is estimated by maximum likehood from $\mathcal{S}$;
2. We draw from another sample $\mathcal{S}^*$, and with replacement, R samples $\mathcal{S}^*_{\tilde{n}^*,r}$ ($r = 1,\ldots,R$) of size $\tilde{n}^* \in N$ where N denotes a set of sample sizes;
3. $\boldsymbol{\beta}^*$ is then estimated by the ML estimate $\hat{\boldsymbol{\beta}}^*_{\tilde{n}^*,r}$ for each sample $\mathcal{S}^*_{\tilde{n}^*,r}$ and for each available model;

4. For each estimate $\hat{\beta}^*_{\tilde{n}^*,r}$, the error rate $e_{\tilde{n}^*,r}$ is estimated from the corresponding unused remaining sample $\mathcal{S}^* \backslash \mathcal{S}^*_{\tilde{n}^*,r}$;

5. Finally, the mean error rate $\bar{e}_{\tilde{n}^*} = R^{-1} \sum_{r=1}^{R} e_{\tilde{n}^*,r}$ is displayed for all $\tilde{n}^*$ values of N and for four models of particular interest: Model selected by BIC, model of lowest error rate, most complex model ($\delta_k \Lambda_k$), simplest model ($0I$).

Thus samples $\mathcal{S}^*_{\tilde{n}^*,r}$ will act as many samples $\mathcal{S}^*$ of different sizes, allowing to study the effect of $\tilde{n}^*$ on each model error rate.

Biology: Continuous covariates and two groups The data set has been already described in Subsection 2.1. We retain *borealis* subspecies as the data set $\mathcal{S}$ ($n = 206$) and *edwardsii* subspecies as the data set $\mathcal{S}^*$ (size $n^* = 92$). Both samples share both common biometrical features ($d = 5$) and common group meaning males/females ($K = 2$). All data are displayed in Figure 2(a) through the first two PCA axes and result of the previous design experiment process, with $N = \{10, 11, 12, \ldots, 40\}$ and $R = 300$, is displayed in Figure 2(b).

In this example, both samples $\mathcal{S}$ and $\mathcal{S}^*$ are so different that the simplest model leads to

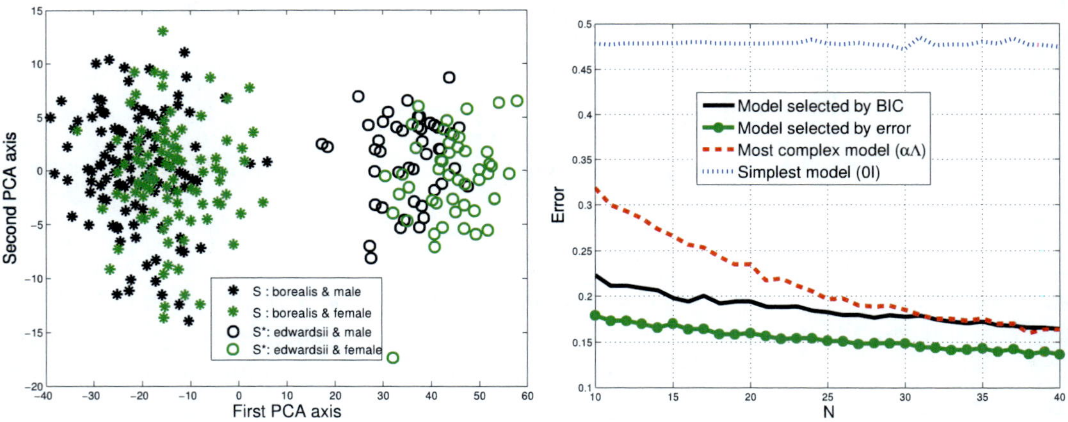

(a) (b)

Figure 2. Birds: (a) Data on the first two PCA axes, (b) mean of the error rate $\bar{e}_{\tilde{n}^*}$ for four models of particular interest.

a very high error rate with subsamples $\mathcal{S}^*_{\tilde{n}^*,r}$ whatever be the sample size $\tilde{n}^*$. As expected, the more complex model is poorly efficient for small values of $\tilde{n}^*$ but it improves when $\tilde{n}^*$ significantly increases. The intermediate model retained by the BIC criterion allows to obtain not only a lower error rate that these too extreme models but also shows a better error rate stability through the values of $\tilde{n}^*$.

Marketing: Categorical covariates and three groups The IncomeESL data set originates from an example in the book [17]. The data set is an extract from this survey. It consists of 8993 instances (obtained from the original data set with 9409 instances, by removing those observations with the annual income missing) with 14 categorical (factors and ordered factors) demographic attributes. It provides from questionnaires containing

502 questions which were filled out by shopping mall customers in the San Francisco Bay area in 1987.

We removed cases with missing values and divided the whole data set into two data sets according to the gender: $\mathcal{S}$ and $\mathcal{S}^*$ respectively correspond to males ($n = 3067$) and females ($n^* = 3809$). In each sample, three groups ($K = 3$) of annual income of households are considered as the response variable: Low income (Less than \$19,999), average income (\$20,000 to \$39,999) and high income (\$40,000 or more). The goal is to predict the annual income of household from the $d = 12$ remaining categorical covariates of two or more modalities and corresponding to demographic attributes. Figure 3(a) displays the first two MCA axes and result of the previous design experiment process, with $N = \{100, 200, 300, \ldots, 1500\}$ and $R = 50$, is displayed in Figure 3(b).

Again, we can see both a nice error rate stability and a low error rate of the intermediate

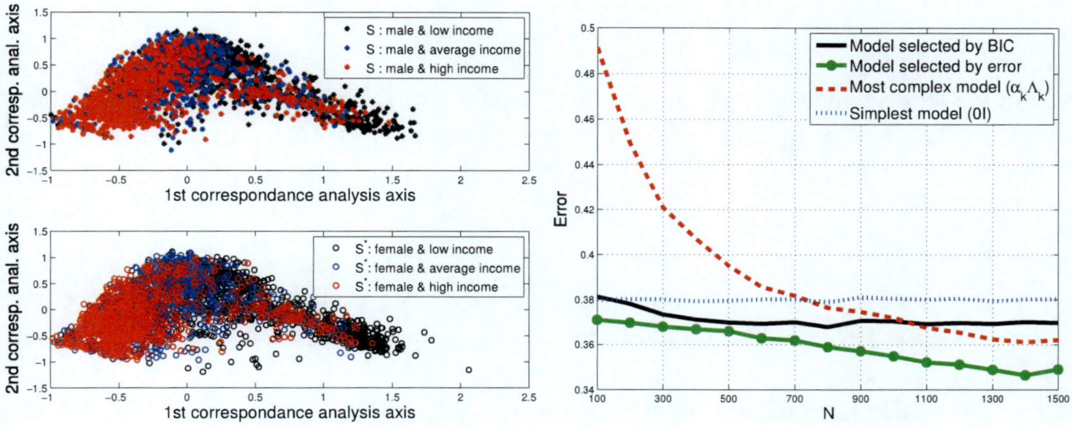

(a) (b)

Figure 3. Birds: (a) Data on the first two MCA axes, (b) mean of the error rate $\bar{e}_{\tilde{n}^*}$ for four models of particular interest.

model retained by the BIC criterion through the values of $\tilde{n}^*$. The simplest model is here more challenging than in the previous biological example since income difference between males and females exists but is quite moderate. A large sample size $\tilde{n}^*$ is required for obtaining good results for the complex model. Thus, the new models act as powerful adaptive challengers for standard models.

3. Parametric transfer learning in regression

Linear regression and mixture of regressions are two very popular techniques to establish a relationship between a quantitative response $y \in \mathcal{Y} = \mathbb{R}$ variable and one or several explanatory variables x. However, as in the classification context, most of the regression methods assume the absence of evolution in the modeled phenomenon between the training and the prediction stages. This section presents parametric transformation models which allows both regression models to deal with evolving populations.

3.1. Linear regression

Linear regression assumes that the response variable $Y \in \mathbb{R}$ can be linked to the explanatory variables $\boldsymbol{x} \in \mathbb{R}^d$ though the relation:

$$Y = \sum_{j=0}^{p} \beta_j \psi_j(\boldsymbol{x}) + \varepsilon,$$

where the residuals $\varepsilon \sim \mathcal{N}(0, \sigma^2)$ are independent, $\boldsymbol{\beta} = (\beta_0, \beta_1, \ldots, \beta_p)' \in \mathbb{R}^{p+1}$ are the regression parameters, $\psi_0(\boldsymbol{x}) = 1$ and $(\psi_j)_{1 \leq j \leq p} : \mathbb{R}^d \to \mathbb{R}$ is a basis of regression functions. The regression functions can be for instance the identity, polynomial functions or splines functions [17]. Let us notice that the usual linear regression occurs when $d = p$ and $\psi_j(\boldsymbol{x}) = x_j$ for $j = 1, \ldots, d$. This model is equivalent to the distributional assumption:

$$Y_{|\mathbf{X}=\boldsymbol{x}} \sim \mathcal{N}(g(\boldsymbol{x}, \boldsymbol{\beta}), \sigma^2),$$

where the regression function $g(\boldsymbol{x}, \boldsymbol{\beta}) = \sum_{j=0}^{p} \beta_j \psi_j(\boldsymbol{x})$ is defined as the conditional expectation $E[Y|\boldsymbol{x}]$. Notice that the regression function can be also written in a matrix form as follows:

$$Y = \boldsymbol{\beta}' \Psi(\boldsymbol{x}) + \varepsilon, \tag{10}$$

where $\Psi(\boldsymbol{x}) = (1, \psi_1(\boldsymbol{x}), \ldots, \psi_p(\boldsymbol{x}))'$.

Learning such a model from a training sample $\mathcal{S} = (\mathbf{x}, \mathbf{y})$ is usually straightforward and relies on ordinary least square (OLS) estimation.

3.1.1. Transfer learning for linear regression

Let us now assume that the regression parameters $\boldsymbol{\beta}$ have been estimated in a preliminary study by using a sample $\mathcal{S}$ of the source population Ω, and that a new regression model has to be adjusted on a new sample $\mathcal{S}^* = (\mathbf{x}^*, \mathbf{y}^*)$, measured on the same explanatory variables but arising from another population Ω^* and for which n^* is assumed to be quite small. The difference between Ω and Ω^* can be for instance geographical or temporal as described in examples of this chapter introduction. The new regression model for Ω^* can be classically written:

$$Y^*_{|\mathbf{X}^*=\boldsymbol{x}^*} \sim \mathcal{N}(\boldsymbol{\beta}^{*\prime} \Psi^*(\boldsymbol{x}^*), \sigma^{2*}). \tag{11}$$

The statistical transformation model aims therefore to define a link between the regression parameters $\boldsymbol{\beta}$ and $\boldsymbol{\beta}^*$. In order to exhibit a link between both regression functions, we make the following important assumptions:

- $\mathcal{A}_1$: We first postulate that the number of basis functions and the basis functions themselves are the same for both regression models ($p^* = p$ and $\psi_j^* = \psi_j$, $\forall j = 1, \ldots, p$).
- $\mathcal{A}_2$: We also assume that the transformation between $g(\bullet, \boldsymbol{\beta})$ and $g(\bullet, \boldsymbol{\beta}^*)$ applies only on the regression parameters. We therefore define the transformation matrix $\boldsymbol{\Lambda}$ between the regression parameters $\boldsymbol{\beta}$ and $\boldsymbol{\beta}^*$ such that $\boldsymbol{\beta}^* = \boldsymbol{\Lambda}\boldsymbol{\beta}$.

- $\mathcal{A}_3$: We finally assume that the relation between the response variable and a specific covariate in the new population Ω^* only depends on the relation between the response variable and the same covariate in the population Ω. Thus, for $j = 0, \ldots, p$, the regression parameter β_j^* only depends on the regression parameter β_j (*i.e.* Λ is diagonal).

The transformation can be finally written in term of the regression parameters of both models as follows:

$$\beta_j^* = \lambda_j \beta_j \qquad \forall j = 0, \ldots, p, \tag{12}$$

where $\lambda_j \in \mathbb{R}$ is the j-th diagonal element of Λ. As previously, it is possible to make further assumptions on the transformation model to makes it more parsimonious. For instance, we allow some of the parameters λ_j to be equal to 1 (in this case the regression parameters β_j^* are equal to β_j). We also allow some of the parameters λ_j to be equal to a common value, *i.e.* $\lambda_j = \lambda$ for given $0 \leq j \leq d$. We list below some of the possible models as declined in [5].

- Model M_0: $\beta_0^* = \lambda_0 \beta_0$ and $\beta_j^* = \lambda_j \beta_j$, for $j = 1, ..., p$. This model is the most complex model of transformation between the populations Ω and Ω^*. It is equivalent to learn a new regression model from the sample $\mathcal{S}^*$, since there is no constraint on the $p+1$ parameters β_j^* ($j = 0, ..., p$), and the number of free parameters in Λ is consequently $p+1$ as well.

- Model M_1: $\beta_0^* = \beta_0$ and $\beta_j^* = \lambda_j \beta_j$ for $j = 1, ..., p$. This model assumes that both regression models have the same intercept β_0.

- Model M_2: $\beta_0^* = \lambda_0 \beta_0$ and $\beta_j^* = \lambda \beta_j$ for $j = 1, ..., p$. This model assumes that the intercept of both regression models differ by the scalar λ_0 and all the other regression parameters differ by the same scalar λ.

- Model M_3: $\beta_0^* = \lambda \beta_0$ and $\beta_j^* = \lambda \beta_j$ for $j = 1, ..., p$. This model assumes that all the regression parameters of both regression models differ by the same scalar λ.

- Model M_4: $\beta_0^* = \beta_0$ and $\beta_j^* = \lambda \beta_j$ for $j = 1, ..., p$. This model assumes that both regression models have the same intercept β_0 and all the other regression parameters differ by the same scalar λ.

- Model M_5: $\beta_0^* = \lambda_0 \beta_0$ and $\beta_j^* = \beta_j$ for $j = 1, ..., p$. This model assumes that both regression models have the same parameters except the intercept.

- Model M_6: $\beta_0^* = \beta_0$ and $\beta_j^* = \beta_j$ for $j = 1, ..., p$. This model assumes that both populations Ω and Ω^* have the same regression model.

The numbers of parameters to estimate for these transformation models are presented in Table 7. The choice of this family is arbitrary and motivated by the will of the authors to treat similarly all the covariates in this general discussion. However, in practical applications, we encourage the practicionners to consider some additional transformation models specifically designed to his application and motivated by his prior knowledge on the subject.
The estimation of the parameters β^* can be deduced from the estimation of the link parameters Λ. Least square estimators for the models M_1 to M_5 are derived in [5].

Table 7. Number of parameters to estimate for the transfer learning models in the linear regression case

Model	M_0	M_1	M_2	M_3	M_4	M_5	M_6
β_0^* is assumed to be	$\lambda_0\beta_0$	β_0	$\lambda_0\beta_0$	$\lambda\beta_0$	β_0	$\lambda_0\beta_0$	β_0
β_i^* is assumed to be	$\lambda_i\beta_i$	$\lambda_i\beta_i$	$\lambda\beta_i$	$\lambda\beta_i$	$\lambda\beta_i$	β_i	β_i
Number of parameters	$p+1$	p	2	1	1	1	0

3.1.2. Biological application

A biological dataset is considered here to highlight the ability of our approach to deal with real data. The *hellung* dataset[1], collected by P. Hellung-Larsen, reports the growth conditions of *Tetrahymena* cells. The data arise from two groups of cell cultures: Cells with and without glucose added to the growth medium. For each group, the average cell diameter (in μm) and the cell concentration (count per ml) were recorded. The cell concentrations of both groups were set to the same value at the beginning of the experiment and it is expected that the presence of glucose in the medium affects the growth of the cell diameter. In the sequel, cells with glucose will be considered as the source population Ω ($n = 32$ observations) whereas cells without glucose will be considered as the target population Ω^* (between $n^* = 11$ to 19 observations).

In order to fit a regression model on the cell group with glucose, the PRESS criterion was used to select the most appropriate basis function. It results that a 3rd degree polynomial function is the most adapted model for these data and this specific basis function will be used for all methods in this experiment. The goal of this experiment is to compare the stability and the effectiveness of the usual OLS regression method with our adaptive linear regression models according to the size of the Ω^* training dataset. For this, 4 different training datasets are used: All Ω^* observations (19 obs.), all Ω^* observations for which the concentration is smaller than 4×10^5 (17 obs.), smaller than 2×10^5 (14 obs.) and smaller than 1×10^5 (11 obs.). In order to evaluate the prediction ability of the different methods, we compute for these 4 different sizes of training dataset the PRESS criterion [1], which represents the mean squared prediction error computed on a cross-validation scheme. This criterion is one of the most often used for model selection in regression analysis, and we encourage its use when it is computationally feasible. In addition, the MSE value (Mean Square Error) on the whole Ω^* dataset is also computed.

Figure 4 illustrates the effect of the training set size on the prediction ability of the studied regression methods. The panels of Figure 4 displays the curve of the usual OLS regression method (M_0) in addition to the curves of the 5 transfer learning models (models M_1 to M_5) for different sizes of the training set (the blue zones indicate the ranges of the observations of Ω^* used for training the models). The model M_6 which is equivalent to the usual OLS regression method on the population Ω is also displayed. The first remark suggested by these results is that the most complex models, OLS (M_0) and M_1, appear to be very unstable in such a situation where the number of training observations is small. Secondly, the model M_4 is more stable but its main assumption (same intercept as the regression model of Ω) seems to be an overly strong constraint and stops it from fitting correctly the

[1]The hellung dataset is available in the ISwR package for R.

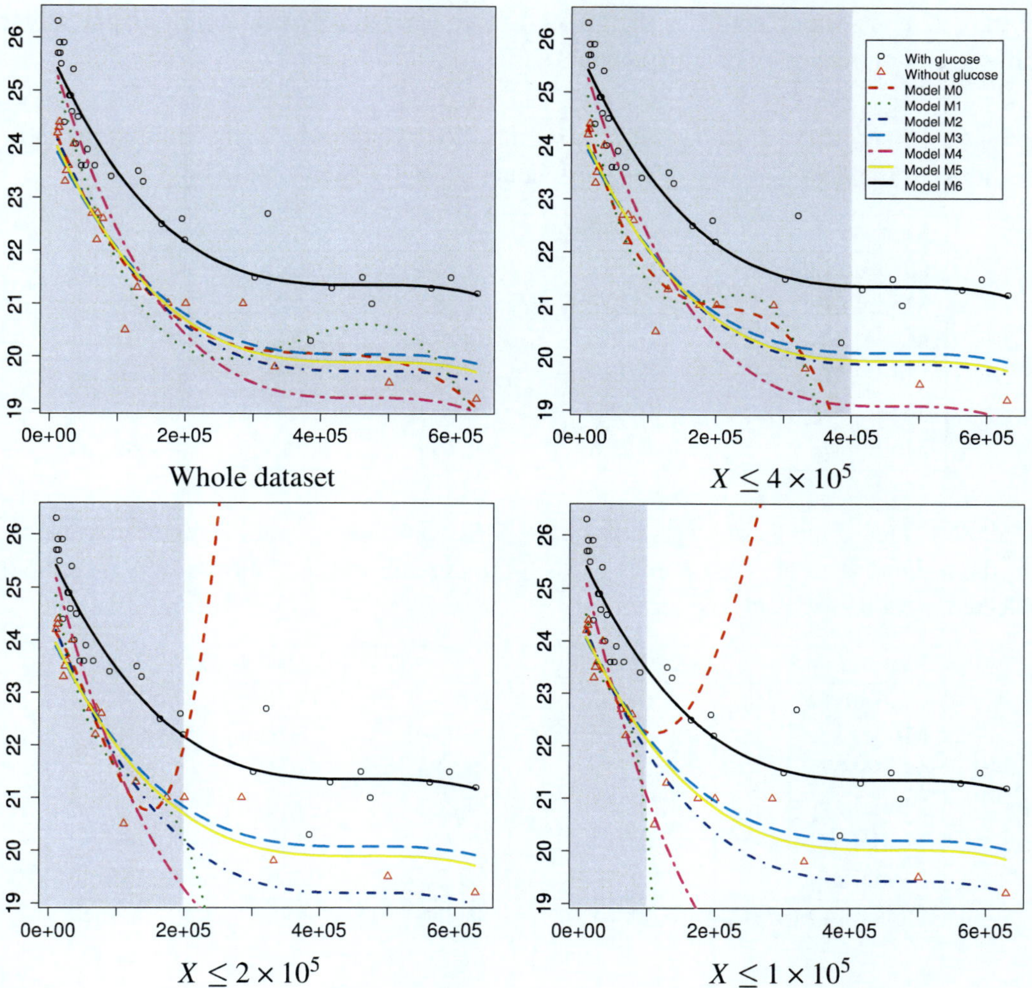

Figure 4. Effect of the learning set size on the prediction ability of the studied regression methods for the *hellung* dataset. The blue zones correspond to the parts of the observations of Ω^* used for learning the models.

data. Finally, the models M_2, M_3 and M_5 turn out to be very stable and flexible enough to correctly model the target population Ω^* even with very few observations. This visual interpretation of the experiment is confirmed by the numerical results presented in Tables 8 and 9. These tables respectively report the value of the PRESS criterion and the MSE associated to the studied regression methods for the different sizes of training dataset. Table 8 confirms clearly that the most stable, and therefore appropriate, model for estimating the transformation between populations Ω and Ω^* is the model M_5. Another interesting conclusion is that both models M_2 and M_3 obtained very low PRESS values as well. These predictions of the model stability appear to be satisfying since the comparison of Tables 8 and 9 shows that the model selected by the PRESS criterion is always an efficient model for prediction. Indeed, Table 9 shows that the most efficient models in practice are the models M_2 and M_5 which are the "preferred" models by PRESS. These two models consider a shift of the intercept, which confirms the guess that we can have by examining graphically the dataset, and moreover by quantifying this shift.

Table 8. Effect of the learning set size on the PRESS criterion of the studied regression methods for the *hellung* dataset. The best values of each column are in bold

Method	whole dataset	$X \leq 4\times10^5$	$X \leq 2\times10^5$	$X \leq 1\times10^5$
OLS on Ω^* (M_0)	0.897	0.364	0.432	0.303
Model M_1	3.332	0.283	2.245	0.344
Model M_2	0.269	0.294	0.261	0.130
Model M_3	0.287	0.271	0.289	0.133
Model M_4	0.859	1.003	0.756	0.517
Model M_5	**0.256**	**0.259**	**0.255**	**0.124**

Table 9. Effect of the learning set size on the MSE value of the studied regression methods for the *hellung* dataset. Best values of each column are in bold and the stars indicate the selected models by the PRESS criterion

Method	whole dataset	$X \leq 4\times10^5$	$X \leq 2\times10^5$	$X \leq 1\times10^5$
OLS on Ω^* (M_0)	0.195	47.718	4.5×10^3	145.846
Model M_1	0.524	164.301	2.3×10^3	5.9×10^5
Model M_2	**0.218**	**0.226**	0.304	**0.245**
Model M_3	0.258	0.262	0.259	0.290
Model M_4	0.791	0.796	1.472	3.046
Model M_5	*0.230	*0.233	***0.230**	*0.246
OLS on Ω (M_6)	2.388	2.388	2.388	2.388

As it could be expected, the advantage of adaptive linear models makes particularly sense when the number of observations of the target population is limited and this happens frequently in real situations due to censorship or to technical constraints (experimental cost, scarcity,...).

3.2. Mixture of regressions

The mixture of regressions, introduced by [15] as the switching regression model and also named clusterwise linear regression model in [18], is a popular regression model for modeling complex systems for which the linear regression model is not flexible enough. In particular, the switching regression model is often used in Economics for modeling phenomena with different phases. Figure 5 illustrates such a situation.

This model assumes that the dependent variable $Y \in \mathcal{Y} = \mathbb{R}$ can be linked to a covariate $\tilde{\boldsymbol{x}} = (1, \boldsymbol{x}) \in \mathbb{R}^{d+1}$ by one of K possible regression models:

$$Y = \boldsymbol{\beta}_k' \Psi(\tilde{\boldsymbol{x}}) + \sigma_k \varepsilon,\ k = 1, ..., K$$

with mixing proportions $\pi_1, \ldots, \pi_K$, where $\varepsilon \sim \mathcal{N}(0,1)$, $\boldsymbol{\beta}_k = (\beta_{k0}, ..., \beta_{kd}) \in \{\boldsymbol{\beta}_1, \ldots, \boldsymbol{\beta}_K\}$ is the regression parameter vector in $\mathbb{R}^{d+1}$ and where $\sigma_k^2 \in \{\sigma_1^2, \ldots, \sigma_K^2\}$ is the residual

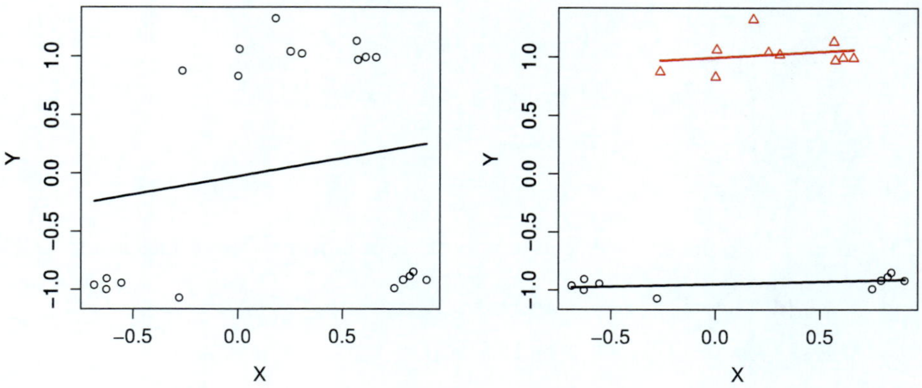

Figure 5. Modelling of a two-state phenomena with the linear regression model (left) and the regression mixture model (right).

variance. The conditional density distribution of Y given $\tilde{\boldsymbol{x}}$ is therefore:

$$f(y|\tilde{\boldsymbol{x}};\boldsymbol{\theta}) = \sum_{k=1}^{K} \pi_k f_k(y; \boldsymbol{\beta}_k^t \Psi(\tilde{\boldsymbol{x}}), \sigma_k^2),$$

where $f_k(\bullet; \boldsymbol{\beta}_k^t \Psi(\tilde{\boldsymbol{x}}), \sigma_k^2)$ is the univariate Gaussian density of mean $\boldsymbol{\beta}_k^t \Psi(\boldsymbol{x})$ and variance σ_k^2. We have also noted $\boldsymbol{\theta} = ((\pi_k, \boldsymbol{\beta}_k, \sigma_k^2) : k = 1, \ldots, K)$. For such a model, the prediction of y for a new observed covariate $\tilde{\boldsymbol{x}}$ is usually carried out in two steps: First the component membership of the data is estimated by the MAP rule following the same principle as in (1) and then y is predicted using the selected regression model.

3.2.1. Transfer learning for mixture of regressions

We make the same assumptions $\mathcal{A}_1$ to $\mathcal{A}_3$ as in the linear regression case and we assume in addition that each mixture is assumed to have the same number of components (*i.e.* $K^* = K$). Conditionally to an observation $\boldsymbol{x}$ of the covariates, we would like to exhibit a distributional relationship between the dependent variables of the same mixture component from available samples $\mathcal{S} = (\mathbf{x}, \mathbf{y})$ and $\mathcal{S}^* = (\mathbf{x}^*, \mathbf{y}^*)$. Let $\boldsymbol{\beta}_k$ and $\boldsymbol{\beta}_k^*$ $(1 \leq k \leq K)$ be respectively the parameters of the mixture regression models in the source and the target populations Ω and Ω^* respectively. [5] assume that the distributional relationship consists of a the following parametric link between the regression parameters of both populations:

$$\boldsymbol{\beta}_k^* = \Lambda_k \boldsymbol{\beta}_k, \text{ where } \Lambda_k = \mathrm{diag}(\lambda_{k0}, \lambda_{k1}, \ldots, \lambda_{kd}) \quad \text{and} \quad \sigma_k^* \text{ is free,}$$

where $\mathrm{diag}(\lambda_{k0}, \lambda_{k1}, \ldots, \lambda_{kd})$ is the diagonal matrix containing $(\lambda_{k0}, \lambda_{k1}, \ldots, \lambda_{kd})$ on its diagonal. In order to introduce parsimony some constraints are put on Λ_k and σ_k^*. Such defined parsimonious models include many of the situations that may be encountered in practice:

- MM_1 assumes both populations are the same: $\Lambda_k = I_d$ is the identity matrix ($\sigma_k^* = \sigma_k$),

- MM_2 models assume the link between both populations is covariate and mixture component independent:
  - MM_{2a} : $\lambda_{k0} = 1$, $\lambda_{kj} = \lambda$ and $\sigma_k^* = \lambda\sigma_k \quad \forall 1 \leq j \leq d$,
  - MM_{2b} : $\lambda_{k0} = \lambda$, $\lambda_{kj} = 1$ and $\sigma_k^* = \sigma_k \quad \forall 1 \leq j \leq d$,
  - MM_{2c} : $\Lambda_k = \lambda I_d$ and $\sigma_k^* = \lambda\sigma_k$,
  - MM_{2d} : $\lambda_{k0} = \lambda_0$, $\lambda_{kj} = \lambda_1$ and $\sigma_k^* = \lambda_1\sigma_k \quad \forall 1 \leq j \leq d$,
- MM_3 models assume the link between both populations is covariate independent:
  - MM_{3a} : $\lambda_{k0} = 1$, $\lambda_{kj} = \lambda_k$ and $\sigma_k^* = \lambda_k\sigma_k \quad \forall 1 \leq j \leq d$,
  - MM_{3b} : $\lambda_{k0} = \lambda_k$, $\lambda_{kj} = 1$ and $\sigma_k^* = \sigma_k \quad \forall 1 \leq j \leq d$,
  - MM_{3c} : $\Lambda_k = \lambda_k I_d$ and $\sigma_k^* = \lambda_k\sigma_k$,
  - MM_{3d} : $\lambda_{k0} = \lambda_{k0}$, $\lambda_{kj} = \lambda_{k1}$ and $\sigma_k^* = \lambda_{k1}\sigma_k \quad \forall 1 \leq j \leq d$,
- MM_4 models assume the link between both populations is mixture component independent (σ_k^* free):
  - MM_{4a} : $\lambda_{k0} = 1$ and $\lambda_{kj} = \lambda_j \quad \forall 1 \leq j \leq d$,
  - MM_{4b} : $\Lambda_k = \Lambda$ with Λ a diagonal matrix,
- MM_5 assumes Λ_k is unconstrained, which leads to estimate the mixture regression model for Ω^* by using only $\mathcal{S}^*$ (σ_k^* free).

Moreover, the mixing proportions are allowed to be the same in each population or to be different. In the latter case, they consequently have to be estimated using the sample $\mathcal{S}^*$. Corresponding notations for the models are respectively $\pi MM_\bullet$ when the mixing proportions π_k^* of Ω^* have to be estimated and $MM_\bullet$ when the have not. Table 10 gives the number of parameters to estimate for each model. If the mixing proportions are different from Ω to Ω^*, $K-1$ parameters to estimate must be added to these values.

Table 10. Number of parameters to estimate for the transfer learning models in the regression mixture case

Model	MM_1	MM_{2a-c}	MM_{2d}	MM_{3a-c}	MM_{3d}	MM_{4a}	MM_{4b}	MM_5
Param. nb.	0	1	2	K	$2K$	$d+K$	$d+K+1$	$K(d+2)$

Model inference The estimation of the link parameters is carried out by ML using a missing data approach *via* the EM algorithm [11]. Indeed, we do not know from which component of the mixture arises each observation $(\boldsymbol{x}_i, y_i)$ or also each observation $(\boldsymbol{x}_i^*, y_i^*)$. This technique is certainly the most popular approach for inference in mixtures of regressions (MCMC approaches can be also used, see [6]). More details on the EM algorithm for the link parameter estimation can be found in [6]. Then, by plug-in, it provides an estimate $\hat{\boldsymbol{\theta}}^*$ of $\boldsymbol{\theta}^*$.

Prediction rule Once the model parameters have been estimated, the prediction $\hat{y}^*$ of the response variable corresponding to an observation $\boldsymbol{x}^*$ of X is obtained by a two step procedure. First, the component membership of $\boldsymbol{x}^*$ is estimated by the MAP rule. Then, $\hat{y}^*$ is predicted using the kth regression model of the mixture:

$$\hat{y}^* = \hat{\boldsymbol{\beta}}_k^{*\prime}\Psi(\tilde{\boldsymbol{x}}^*).$$

Model selection In order to select among the differents transfer learning models the most appropriate model of transformation between the populations Ω and Ω^* , we propose to use two well-known criteria, already presented: PRESS and BIC. Let us recall that, for both criteria, the most adapted model is the one with the smallest criterion value.

3.2.2. Economic-environmental application

In this experiment, the link between CO_2 emission and gross national product (GNP) of various countries is investigated. The sources of the data are *The official United Nations site for the Millennium Development Goals Indicators* and the *World Development Indicators of the World Bank.* Figure 6 plots the CO_2 emission per capita *versus* the logarithm of GNP per capita for 111 countries, in 1980 (left) and 1999 (right).

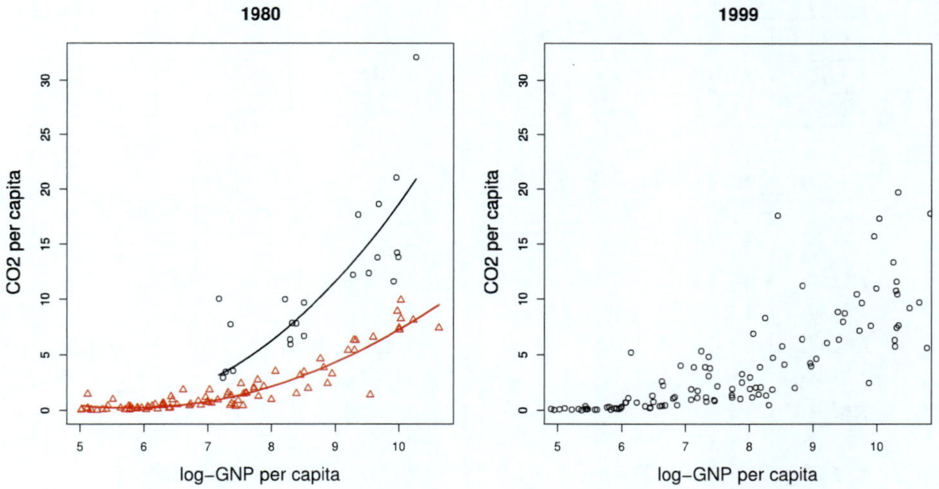

Figure 6. Emission of CO_2 per capita *versus* GNP per capita in 1980 (left) and 1999 (right).

A mixture of second order polynomial regressions seems to be particularly well adapted to fit these data and will be used in the following. Let remark that regression model with heteroscedasticity could also be appropriated for such data, but these kinds of models are out of the topic of the present work. For the 1980's data, two groups of countries are easily distinguishable: A first minority group (about 25% of the whole sample) is made of countries for which a grow in the GNP is linked to a high grow of the CO_2 emission, whereas the second group (about 75%) seems to have more environmental political orientations. As pointed out by [20], the study of such data could be particularly useful for countries with low GNP in order to clarify in which development path they are embarking. This country discrimination in two groups is more difficult to obtain on the 1999's data: It seems that countries which had high CO_2 emission in 1980 have adopted a more environmental development than in the past, and a two-component mixture regression model could be more difficult to exhibit.

Table 11. MSE on the whole 1999's sample, PRESS and BIC criterion for the 10 parametric transfer learning models (πMM_{2a} to πMM_{4b}), usual regression model (UR) and classical regressions mixture model (MR), for 4 sizes of the 1999's sample: 33, 55, 77 and 111 (whole sample). Lower BIC, PRESS and MSE values for each sample size are in bold character

30% of the 1999's data ($n^* = 33$)

model	BIC	PRESS	MSE
πMM_{2a}	13.09	**3.38**	3.40
πMM_{2b}	12.73	3.89	**3.32**
πMM_{2c}	12.79	5.48	3.68
πMM_{2d}	11.54	4.99	3.73
πMM_{3a}	12.14	4.20	3.76
πMM_{3b}	11.72	4.87	4.00
πMM_{3c}	**11.50**	5.09	3.86
πMM_{3d}	22.83	5.52	3.64
πMM_{4a}	18.72	5.15	4.01
πMM_{4b}	22.01	6.21	5.04
UR	27.08	7.46	7.66
MR	32.89	5.54	5.11

50% of the 1999's data ($n^* = 55$)

model	BIC	PRESS	MSE
πMM_{2a}	**10.18**	4.11	3.44
πMM_{2b}	13.54	3.73	3.37
πMM_{2c}	13.89	4.25	3.45
πMM_{2d}	22.35	4.38	4.80
πMM_{3a}	12.00	3.84	4.49
πMM_{3b}	12.00	4.47	3.86
πMM_{3c}	17.53	3.97	**3.28**
πMM_{3d}	25.39	4.77	3.67
πMM_{4a}	20.65	**3.68**	3.44
πMM_{4b}	24.92	5.57	4.19
UR	20.87	7.95	7.21
MR	39.69	4.82	4.77

70% of the 1999's data ($n^* = 77$)

model	BIC	PRESS	MSE
πMM_{2a}	14.76	**3.65**	3.35
πMM_{2b}	14.73	3.91	3.39
πMM_{2c}	**14.53**	4.49	3.53
πMM_{2d}	18.90	4.30	3.72
πMM_{3a}	18.84	4.33	3.85
πMM_{3b}	18.80	4.40	3.85
πMM_{3c}	18.81	4.41	3.26
πMM_{3d}	27.05	3.91	**3.17**
πMM_{4a}	22.29	5.25	4.00
πMM_{4b}	26.55	4.92	4.03
UR	22.08	8.00	7.10
MR	43.91	5.06	3.33

($n^* = 111$)

model	BIC	PRESS	MSE
πMM_{2a}	15.51	4.78	3.32
πMM_{2b}	15.44	3.81	3.37
πMM_{2c}	**15.39**	4.84	3.47
πMM_{2d}	20.05	4.45	3.59
πMM_{3a}	20.18	4.29	3.79
πMM_{3b}	20.03	4.38	3.77
πMM_{3c}	20.05	3.94	3.10
πMM_{3d}	29.37	4.08	3.34
πMM_{4a}	23.98	4.21	4.13
πMM_{4b}	28.58	5.21	4.52
UR	23.62	7.53	6.99
MR	47.19	**3.66**	**2.89**

In order to help this distinction, parametric transfer learning models are used to estimate the mixture regression model on the 1999's data. The ten parametric transfer learning models, with free component proportions π_k^*, πMM_{2a} to πMM_{4b}, classical mixture of second order polynomial regressions with two components (MR) and usual second order polynomial regression (UR) are considered. Different sample size of the 1999's data are tested: 30%, 50%, 70% and 100% of the $\mathcal{S}^*$ size ($n^* = 111$). The experiments have been repeated 20 times in order to average the results. Table 11 summarizes these results where MSE corresponds to the mean square error. In this application, the total number of available data in the 1999 population is not sufficiently large to separate them into two training and test samples. For this reason, MSE is computed on the whole $\mathcal{S}^*$ sample, even though a part of it has been used for the training (from 30% for the first experiment to 100% for the last one). Consequently, MSE is a significant indicator of predictive ability of the model when 30% and 50% of the whole dataset are used as training set since 70% and 50% of the samples used to compute the MSE remain independent from the training stage. However, MSE is a less significant indicator of predictive ability for the two last experiments and the PRESS should be preferred in these situations as indicator of predictive ability.

Table 11 first allows to remark that the 1999's data are actually made of two components as in the 1980's data since both PRESS and MSE are better for MR (2 components) than UR (1 component) for all sizes n^* of $\mathcal{S}^*$. This first result validates the assumption that both the reference population Ω and the new population Ω^* have the same number $K = 2$ components, and consequently the use of transfer learning techniques makes sense for this data. Secondly, AMR models turn out to provide very satisfying predictions for all values of n^* and particularly outperforms the other approaches when n^* is relatively small (less than 77 here). Indeed, both BIC, PRESS and MSE testify that the transfer learning models provide better predictions than the other studied methods when n^* is equal to 30%, 50% and 70% of the whole sample. Furthermore, it should be noticed that transfer learning models provide stable results according to variations on n^*. In particular, the models πMM_2 are those which appear the most efficient on this dataset and this means that the link between both populations Ω and Ω^* is mixture component independent.

This application illustrates the interest of combining informations on both past (1980) and present (1999) situations in order to analyse the link between CO_2 emissions and gross national product for several countries in 1999, especially when the number of data for the present situation is not sufficiently large. Moreover, the competition between the parametric transfer learning models is also informative. Effectively, it seems that three models are particularly well adapted to model the link between the 1980's data and those of 1999's data: πMM_{2a}, πMM_{2b} and πMM_{2c}. The particularity of these models is that they consider the same transformation for both classes of countries, which means, conversely to what one might *prima facie* have thought, that all the countries have made an effort to reduce their CO_2 emissions and not only those which had the higher ones.

4. Parametric transfer learning in clustering

4.1. The statistical model

Clustering aims to partition a sample $\mathcal{S} = \mathbf{x}$ of n observed data into K groups. The standard model-based clustering procedure assumes that any observed data $\boldsymbol{x}_i \in \mathcal{S}$ $(i = 1,\ldots,n)$ is i.i.d. drawn from a random vector $\boldsymbol{X}$ of the K-component mixture of parametric distributions $f(\bullet;\boldsymbol{\theta}) = \sum_{k=1}^{K} \pi_k f_k(\bullet;\alpha_k)$. We recall that π_k denotes the mixing proportions of the component k, α_k its parameter and $\boldsymbol{\theta} = \{(\pi_k,\alpha_k) : k = 1,\ldots,K\}$ the whole mixture parameter. It can be assumed equivalently that (i) $\boldsymbol{x}_i$ has been generated by the component $y_i \in \{1,\ldots,K\}$ with probability π_{y_i} and that (ii) the component of origin y_i is a lost information. Thus the vector $\mathbf{y} = (y_1,\ldots,y_n)$ constitutes some hidden data (see [27], p. 7).

The clustering procedure consists in three stages. First, the parameter θ has to be estimated by the ML principle, usually by the mean of an EM algorithm. Second, observed data $\mathbf{x}$ are allocated by the MAP rule to the group corresponding to the highest estimated conditional probability of membership computed at the ML estimate $\hat{\theta}$: See (1) and (2) in this chapter (see also [27] p. 31). Finally, the BIC criterion is commonly used for selecting some parsimonious model and/or the number of clusters (see [14, 30]).

4.2. Gaussian transfer learning and its estimation

Thereafter we aim to partition, in a Gaussian context, not a single sample, but H n^h-samples $S^h = \mathbf{x}^h$ $(h = 1, \ldots, H)$, with $\mathbf{x}^h = (x_1^h, \ldots, x_{n^h}^h)$, described by a set of d continuous variables (so $\mathcal{X} = \mathbb{R}^d$) into K groups each. Thus, in this section, we are no longer limited to two populations, a source one (Ω) and a target one (Ω^*), but we are in a more general situation where H populations $\Omega^1, \ldots, \Omega^H$ are present. Note that all populations will now play a symmetric role (instead of previous discriminant analysis and regression situations), so the concept of "source" and "target" population becomes totally arbitrary and unimportant. In addition, we make the assumptions that (i) the samples share statistical units of same nature, (ii) they are described by identical features and (iii) all researched partitions $\mathbf{y}^a = (y_1^h, \ldots, y_{n^h}^h)$ share the same meaning.

Such situations are numerous and it is easily to exhibit examples through well-known data sets. For instance the Old Faithful geyser located in the Yellowstone National Park (Wyoming, USA) is regularly subject to clustering investigations. Figure 7 displays two samples of the geyser eruptions differing over ten years and described by the same variables: Duration and inter-eruption waiting time interval (in minutes). Some structure of the eruptions is frequently researched within one of these samples, but never by using the whole information that they both provide. Sections 4.3. and 4.4. present also two other situations, the first one in Biology and the second one in Finance, where several samples of identical statistical units described by the same features, have to be clustered into same meaning partitions.

4.2.1. Independent clustering of several populations

Standard Gaussian model-based clustering assumes that each individual x_i^h of the sample $\mathbf{x}^h$ $(h \in \{1, \ldots, H\})$ is i.i.d. drawn from a population Ω^h modelled by a mixture of K normal d-dimensional distributions. In addition, all samples $\mathbf{x}^h$ are mutually independent. The component k is weighted by $\pi_k^h > 0$ $(\sum_{j=1}^K \pi_j^h = 1)$, centered in $\mu_k^h \in \mathbb{R}^d$ with covariance matrix $\Sigma_k^h \in \mathbb{R}^{d \times d}$ (symmetric positive-definite) and $\mathbf{y}^h = (y_1^h, \ldots, y_K^h)$ is the missing response variable indicating the component from which each x_i^h arises. So the mixture Ω^h is entirely parameterized by $\theta^h = \{(\pi_k^h, \mu_k^h, \Sigma_k^h) : k = 1, \ldots, K\}$.

The standard independent procedure considers that the populations Ω^h $(h = 1, \ldots, H)$ are unrelated and so, that the parameters θ^h are algebraically free. Then estimating the whole model parameter $\theta = (\theta^1, \ldots, \theta^H)$ by maximum likelihood, is equivalent to estimating each parameter θ^h independently from the others. Indeed, $\ell(\theta) = \sum_{h=1}^H \ell^h(\theta^h)$ where $\ell(\theta)$ is the log-likelihood of θ computed on the whole observed data $\mathbf{x} = (\mathbf{x}^1, \ldots, \mathbf{x}^H)$, and $\ell^h(\theta^h)$ is the log-likelihood of θ^h computed on the observed data $\mathbf{x}^h$ only. Then, all par-

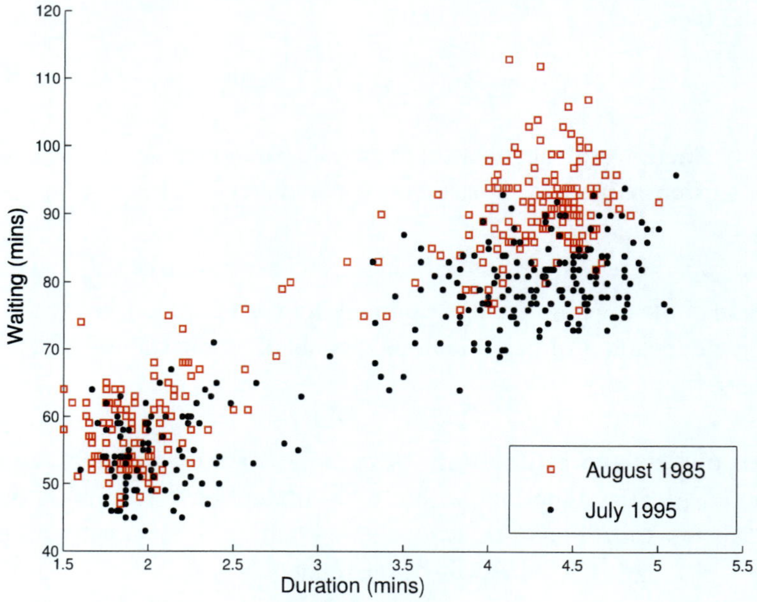

Figure 7. Two samples of Old Faithful geyser eruptions differing over 10 years.

titions $\mathbf{y}^h$ are estimated by performing the MAP rule on observed data $\mathbf{x}^h$ by using the obtained ML estimate of $\boldsymbol{\theta}^h$.

That first standard method proceeds as if the diverse samples to be classified were unrelated and prohibits any transfer learning between the populations. But let us remind that (i) the samples share statistical units of same nature (ii) they are described by the same features and (iii) the groups that have to be discovered consist in a same meaning partition of each sample. The simultaneous clustering method [23] that we present now, formalizes the previous informations by establishing a link between the populations, in order to improve the model fit and the estimated partitions.

4.2.2. Simultaneous clustering of several populations

Let assume that observations of $(\mathbf{x}^h, \mathbf{y}^h)$ are i.i.d. realizations of a random couple $(\boldsymbol{X}^h, Y^h)$. For all $(h,h') \in \{1,\ldots,H\}^2$ and all $k \in \{1,\ldots,K\}$, we suppose that there exist $\boldsymbol{D}_k^{h,h'} \in \mathbb{R}^{d\times d}$ diagonal, regular, positive and $\boldsymbol{b}_k^{h,h'} \in \mathbb{R}^d$ such that:

$$\boldsymbol{X}^{h'}_{|Y^{h'}=k} \stackrel{\mathscr{D}}{=} \boldsymbol{D}_k^{h,h'} \boldsymbol{X}^h_{|Y^h=k} + \boldsymbol{b}_k^{h,h'}. \tag{13}$$

Some arguments for justifying this affine form have been already discussed in Section 2.1.2. and can be also find in [23]. Note that the condition that $\boldsymbol{D}_k^{h,h'}$ be positive is imposed for identifiability reasons. This positivity involves that the correlation sign of any couple of conditional variables keeps unchanged through the populations. That constraint seems to be realistic in many experimental situations.

Equivalently to (13), the following parametric link can be established between populations. Whatever are k, h, h', there exists some diagonal positive-definite matrix $\boldsymbol{D}_k^{h,h'} \in$

$\mathbb{R}^{d\times d}$ and some vector $\boldsymbol{b}_k^{h,h'} \in \mathbb{R}^d$, such that:

$$\boldsymbol{\Sigma}_k^{h'} = \boldsymbol{D}_k^{h,h'} \boldsymbol{\Sigma}_k^h \boldsymbol{D}_k^{h,h'} \text{ and } \boldsymbol{\mu}_k^{h'} = \boldsymbol{D}_k^{h,h'} \boldsymbol{\mu}_k^h + \boldsymbol{b}_k^{h,h'}. \tag{14}$$

Property (14) characterizes henceforward the whole parameter space of $\boldsymbol{\theta}$ and the so-called simultaneous clustering method is based on $\boldsymbol{\theta}$ parameter inference in that so constrained parameter space.

Let us set: $p_k^{h,h'} = \pi_k^{h'}/\pi_k^h$ for all k, h and h'. Then matrices $\boldsymbol{D}_k^{h,h'}$, vectors $\boldsymbol{b}_k^{h,h'}$ and scalars $p_k^{h,h'}$ constitute a whole parametric bond between populations, which is helpful (i) for defining some meaningful parsimonious models of stochastic transformations and (ii) for estimating $\boldsymbol{\theta}$.

Parsimonious models and estimation Several parsimonious models can be considered by combining classical assumptions within each mixture on both mixing proportions and Gaussian parameters (*intrapopulation* models), with meaningful constraints on the link parameters $\boldsymbol{D}_k^{h,h'}$, $\boldsymbol{b}_k^{h,h'}$ and $p_k^{h,h'}$ (*interpopulation* models).
Intrapopulation models. Inspired by standard Gaussian model-based clustering, one can envisage several classical parsimonious models of constraints on the Gaussian mixtures P^h: Their components may be homoscedastic ($\boldsymbol{\Sigma}_k^h = \boldsymbol{\Sigma}^h$) or heteroscedastic, their mixing proportions may be equal ($\pi_k^h = \pi^h$) or free.
Interpopulation models. In the most general case, $\boldsymbol{D}_k^{h,h'}$ matrices are positive-definite and diagonal, $\boldsymbol{b}_k^{h,h'}$ vectors are unconstrained and $p_k^{h,h'}$ scalars are positive. We can also consider component independent situations on $\boldsymbol{D}_k^{h,h'}$ ($\boldsymbol{D}_k^{h,h'} = \boldsymbol{D}^{h,h'}$), on $\boldsymbol{b}_k^{h,h'}$ ($\boldsymbol{b}_k^{h,h'} = \boldsymbol{b}^{h,h'}$) and/or on $p_k^{h,h'}$ ($p_k^{h,h'} = p^{h,h'}$).

Let us mention briefly that some combinations of the previous constraints are not allowed. For example, the mixing proportions cannot be assumed to be homogeneous within each mixture (π^h) and free through the populations ($p_k^{h,h'}$). All allowed combinations of intra and interpopulation models are available in [23]. They constitute a family of Gaussian mixture-based simultaneous clustering models.

Assuming that H samples $\mathcal{S}^1,\ldots,\mathcal{S}^H$ are drawn from the H populations $\Omega^1,\ldots,\Omega^H$, estimation of the model parameter by ML is carried out by the EM algorithm. We refer to [23] for more details.

4.3. Biological application of Gaussian transfer learning

In [32] three seabird subspecies ($H = 3$) of Cory's Shearwaters, differing over their geographical range, are described. *Borealis* (size $n^1 = 206$ individuals, 45% female) are living in the Atlantic Islands (Azores, Canaries, etc.), *diomedea* (size $n^2 = 38$ individuals, 58% female), in Mediterranean Islands (Balearics, Corsica, etc.), and *edwardsii* (size $n^3 = 92$ individuals, 52% female), in Cape Verde Islands. Only the two first subspecies have been considered in Application 2.1.3. Individuals are described in all species by the same five morphological variables ($d = 5$): Culmen (bill length), tarsus, wing and tail lengths, and culmen depth. We aim to cluster each subspecies.

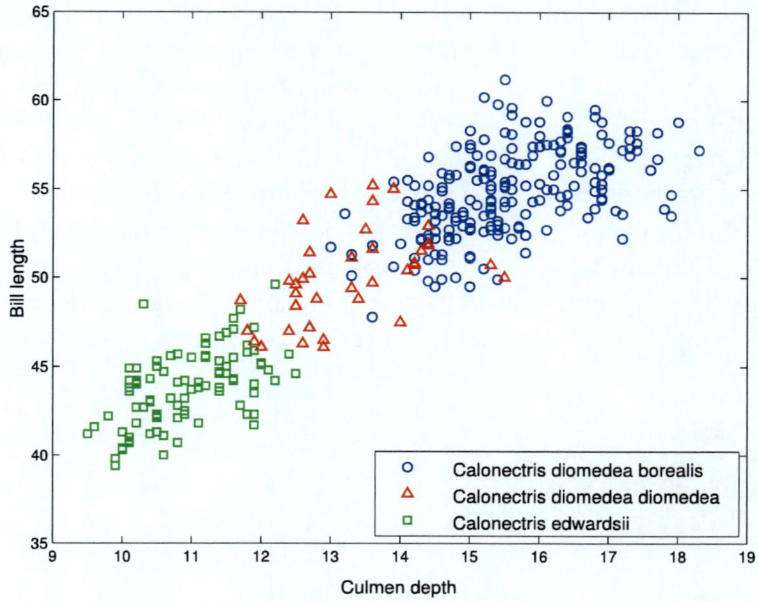

Figure 8. Three samples of Cory's Shearwaters described by identical features.

Figure 8 displays the birds in the plane of the culmen depth and the bill length. Samples seem clearly to arise from three different populations, so three standard independent Gaussian model-based clusterings should be considered. But as all of them arise from the same species *calonectris diomedea*, the researched partitions could be expected to have the same number of clusters with the same partition meaning in each sample. In addition, the three samples are described by the same five morphological features, thus the data set could be suitable for some simultaneous clustering process. As a consequence, it is quite reasonable that both simultaneous and independent clustering compete. The following paragraphs compare the results obtained from simultaneous and independent clustering.

Selecting the number of clusters Table 12 displays the best BIC criterion value among all models for the two clustering strategies. The overall best BIC value (4071.8) is obtained from simultaneous clustering for $K = 2$ groups. This value is widely better than the best BIC obtained from independent clustering ($BIC = 4102.6$). So BIC clearly prefers the simultaneous clustering method and rejects, here, the standard independent clustering method.

Table 12. Best BIC values obtained in clustering the Cory's Shearwaters simultaneously and independently, with different number of clusters

Cluster Number	1	2	3	4
Simultaneous Clustering	4073.3	**4071.8**	4076.7	4082.4
Independent Clustering	4102.6	4139.8	4137.7	4159.6

Determing the gender of birds Retaining the two cluster solution ($\hat{K} = 2$) we propose now to compare the partition estimated in each method with the gender partition of birds (males/females). The error rate associated to the best model of simultaneous clustering (BIC = 4071.8) is 10.71% whereas the best model of independent clustering (BIC = 4139.8) reaches 12.50%. Let us add that 10.71% is also the overall best error rate observed in both methods. So the best model according to BIC (provided by simultaneous clustering) is also the overall best global classifier. Moreover, Figure 9 and the confusion tables in Table 13 (a) and Table 13 (b), highlight the following point: By sexing differently few birds from the independent clustering, the simultaneous method improves not only the global error rate, but also the correlation between the estimated clusters and the bird genders.

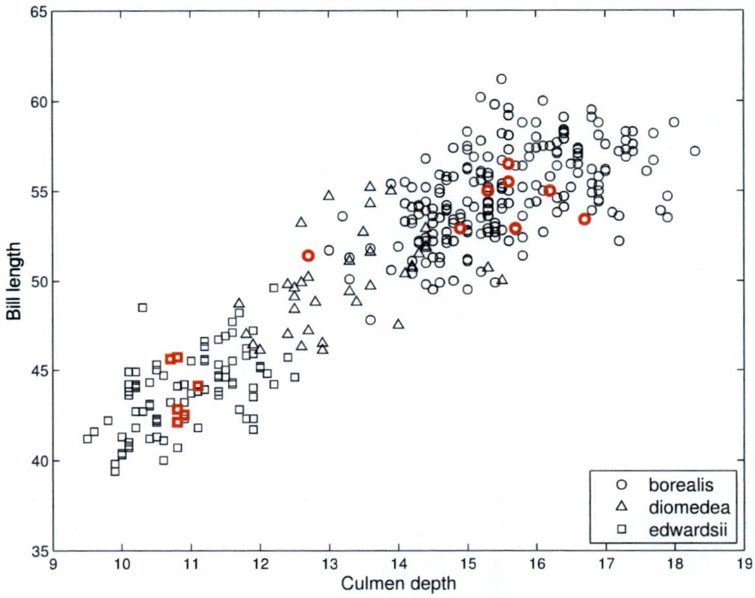

Figure 9. Similarities (in black) and differences (in red) between independent (BIC = 4139.8) and simultaneous clustering (BIC = 4071.8), in sexing each Shearwater sample.

Interpreting the selected model The overall best model (BIC = 4071.8) specifies the following points. Firstly, the matrices $\boldsymbol{\Sigma}_k^h$ are homogeneous on k (every mixture is homoscedastic). So the covariance of any couple of biometrical variables should be the same among males and females (in each subspecies). This assertion makes sense and is realistic for ornithologists. Secondly, $\pi_1^h = \pi_2^h$ whatever is $h \in \{1,2,3\}$. There are as many males than females in *borealis*, *diomedea* and *edwardsii* subspecies. This is realistic, given the gender partition of each sample. So, the two previous points are in accordance with the best model of independent clustering (BIC = 4139.8). In addition, the greater originality of the model provided by simultaneous clustering (BIC = 4071.8) lies in the following point: All transformation parameters $p_k^{h,h'}$, $\boldsymbol{b}_k^{h,h'}$ and $\boldsymbol{D}_k^{h,h'}$ are homogeneous on k. So, simultaneous clustering does not only provide the best model (according to BIC and according to the error

Table 13. Confusion tables obtained by comparing the inferred clusters within each subspecies ($K = 2$ groups) to the sex of the birds

(a) Independent clustering (BIC=4139.8).

		cluster 1	cluster 2
borealis	male	20	93
	female	88	5
diomedea	male	1	15
	female	18	4
edwardsii	male	7	37
	female	43	5

(b) Simultaneous clustering (BIC=4071.8).

		cluster 1	cluster 2
borealis	male	18	95
	female	89	4
diomedea	male	2	14
	female	18	4
edwardsii	male	5	39
	female	45	3

rate), but this model allows also the following interpretation: There exists a mutual stochastic transformation of the males across the subspecies, there exists another transformation of the females, and these two transformations are identical.

4.4. Robust transfer learning and its estimation

As the Gaussian parameters are sensitive to extreme values, normal mixtures may be unsuitable for modeling the data when they are suspected to include noise or outliers. Alternatively, one can assume that the distribution of $\boldsymbol{X}^h$ conditionally to Y_k^h is no more Gaussian but corresponds to a d-dimensional Student's t distribution with degree of freedom $\nu_k^h \in \mathbb{R}_*^+$, location parameter $\boldsymbol{\mu}_k^h \in \mathbb{R}^d$ and (symmetric positive-definite) inner product matrix $\boldsymbol{\Sigma}_k^h \in \mathbb{R}^{d\times d}$ (see [27], chapter 7). We note in this case $\boldsymbol{\theta}^h = \{(\pi_k^h, \boldsymbol{\mu}_k^h, \boldsymbol{\Sigma}_k^h, \nu_k^h) : k = 1,\dots,K\}$ and again $\boldsymbol{\theta} = (\boldsymbol{\theta}^1,\dots,\boldsymbol{\theta}^H)$.

[24] consider several parsimonious models of unlinked t-mixtures: Mixing proportions π_k^h are either free or homogeneous on k, as degrees of freedom ν_k^h and/or inner product matrices $\boldsymbol{\Sigma}_k^h$. Without any other constraint on the Student's parameters, the model at hand involves an independent clustering procedure.

However, the mutual affine transformation of the conditional populations formalized by (13), can also be assumed in this new context of Student's t mixtures. This transformation is justified as in Section 4.2. when: (i) The samples share statistical units of same nature (ii) they are described by identical features and (iii) the expected partitions are about to be identically interpreted. Such an affine mutation of the conditional t-populations implicates that the degrees of freedom ν_k^h are homogeneous on h: $\nu_k^1 =, \dots, = \nu_k^H = \nu_k$. Then interpopulation models are obtained by considering that $\boldsymbol{D}_k^{h,h'}$ matrices, $\boldsymbol{b}_k^{h,h'}$ vectors and/or $p_k^{h,h'}$ scalars are either free or homogeneous on k.

Combining the previous constraints on (i) the intrapopulation parameters π_k^h, ν_k^h, $\boldsymbol{\Sigma}_k^h$ and (ii) the transformation parameters $p_k^{h,h'}$, $\boldsymbol{b}_k^{h,h'}$, $\boldsymbol{D}_k^{h,h'}$, leads to a family of t-mixture-based simultaneous clustering models. As in the Gaussian case some of the proposed constraints cannot be matched and one has to refer to [24] in order to find all allowed combinations of intra and interpopulation models. The estimation of $\boldsymbol{\theta}$ by ML requires a Generalized EM algorithm (see [11]) and details are given again in [24].

Any likelihood-based criterion can help to (i) select a model of independent clustering, (ii) select a model of simultaneous clustering and (iii) determine the best clustering method among the two previous ones. The BIC criterion was used for that purpose in Section 4.2. But BIC reports essentially the adequacy of the model and sometimes at the expense of the interpretability of the associated partition. In order to avoid some spurious components (see [27]) due to the noise within the data, BIC can be replaced by the ICL criterion (see [4]) defined by

$$\mathrm{ICL} = \mathrm{BIC} - 2\sum_{h=1}^{H}\sum_{k=1}^{K}\sum_{\{i:\hat{y}_i^h=k\}} \ln t_k(\boldsymbol{x}_i^h;\hat{\boldsymbol{\theta}}^h),$$

where $\hat{y}_i^h$ denotes the MAP estimate of y_i^h and $t_k(\boldsymbol{x}_i^h;\hat{\boldsymbol{\theta}}^h)$ is the conditional probability of membership of $\boldsymbol{x}_i^h$ to the cluster k (it is a straightforward adaptation of (2)). ICL penalizes the models with strong overlap components, so it provides partitions where the clusters are well-separated and, consequently, easier to interpret. The model with the smallest ICL value has to be retained.

4.5. Economic application of robust transfer learning

In [12] Du Jardin and Séverin display several samples of firms differing over the year and described by the same econometric variables. On two samples from these financial data, suspected by the authors to contain outliers, we propose to compare the simultaneous and the independent clustering strategies both based on t-mixtures. The first sample from 2002 consists of 428 firms (212 bankrupt ones) and the second sample from 2003, of 461 companies (220 bankrupt ones). Both samples are described by four financial ratios: EBITDA/Total Assets, Value Added/Total Sales, Quick Ratio, Accounts Payable/Total Sales. Figure 10 represents the two datasets in the canonical plane: [EBITDA/Total Assets, Quick ratio]. Table 14 displays the best ICL criterion value among all models for simultaneous clustering strategy. We notice that ICL retains a three clusters ($K = 3$) solution.

Table 14. Best ICL values, over all models, obtained in simultaneous and independent clustering with different number of clusters

K	1	2	3	4	5
Simultaneous	−1169.7	−1191.3	**−1202.0**	−1183.4	−1131.3
Independent	−1154.6	**−1163.6**	−1072.1	−1127.7	−1098.3

Table 15 gives the associated confusion table of this obtained partition in comparison to the bankruptcy and healthy specifications. We see that estimated Clusters 1 and 2 are highly correlated respectively to failed and no-failed companies, whereas Cluster 3 is clearly a group where failed and no-failed companies are indistinguishable.

This typology indicates that it is easy to identify very well healthy and non-healthy companies (see Figure 11) for a small number of cases (Clusters 1 and 2 have respectively mixing proportions equal to 0.07 and 0.13) whereas it is expected to be a very hard task for most of them (Cluster 3 has a mixing proportion of 0.80).

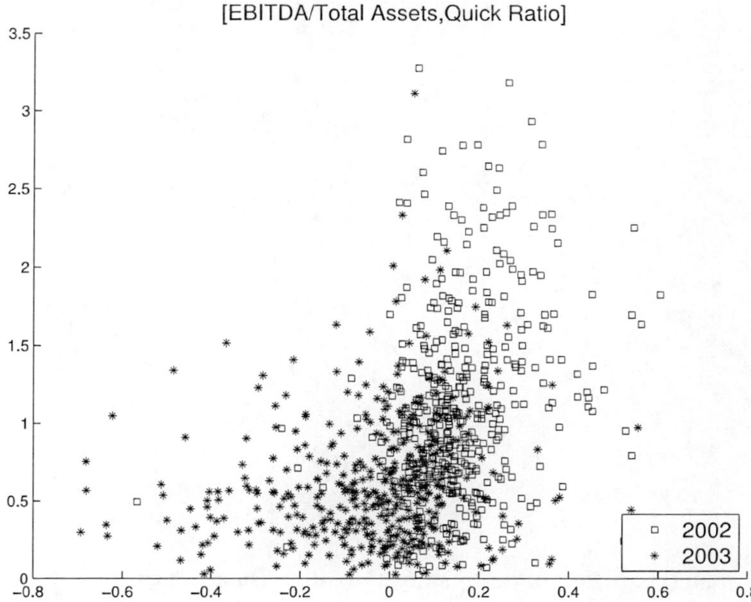

Figure 10. Two samples of companies differing over the year.

Table 15. Confusion table associated to the partition provided by the best simultaneous clustering model retained by ICL

	Cluster 1	Cluster 2	Cluster 3
Healthy	3	94	360
Bankruptcy	56	10	366

In addition, by using t-parameters of each cluster, it is obviously possible to draw a synthetic description of each of them (classical analysis in model-based clustering so not reported here) but we focus on the specificity of simultaneous clustering which provides an information about the group evolution over the years. The retained model (ICL $= -1202.2$) states that every mutation parameter p_k^h, $\boldsymbol{b}_k^{h,h'}$, $\boldsymbol{D}_k^{h,h'}$ is homogeneous on k, that the degrees of freedom ν_k and the inner product matrices Σ_k^h do not depend on k either, and that the reference mixing proportions π_k^1 are free. Then, according to this model: (i) The mixing proportion of each cluster is invariant between 2002 and 2003 and (ii) other cluster features uniformly evolved over the years. More precisely, the associated estimated transition parameters are given by:

$$\begin{aligned} \hat{\boldsymbol{D}}^{1,2} &= \text{diag}(1.12, 0.95, 1.20, 0.93) \\ \hat{\boldsymbol{b}}^{1,2} &= 10^{-3}.(-18.2, 2, -102, -1)', \end{aligned}$$

thus clusters from 2002 and 2003 appear to vary only through the two variables EBITDA/Total Assets and Quick Ratio. This result is meaningful: These two variables report respectively the liquidity and the performance of the firms, which are known to be

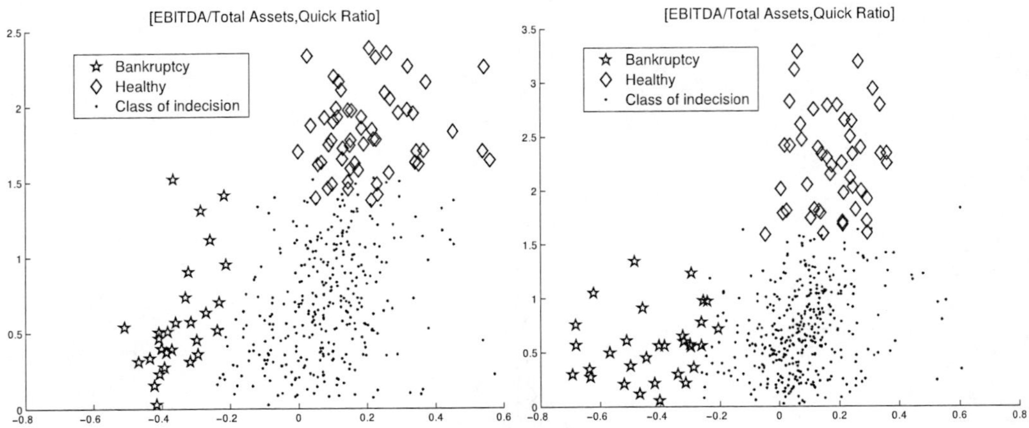

(a) *year* 2002

(b) *year* 2003

Figure 11. Estimated partition of companies (Healthy, Bankruptcy, Indecision) for the two consecutive years (2002, 2003), obtained by a simultaneous t-mixture model-based clustering methodology.

the main features able to predict bankruptcy. Indeed the change of the financial structure is a consequence of the evolution of these two features.

For comparison, Table 14 displays also the best ICL criterion value among all models for independent clustering. We notice now that $K = 2$ clusters are retained and the associated confusion table (Table 16) indicates that estimated clusters bring poor information about the company health in comparison to the three components solution given by simultaneous clustering. In addition, independent clustering does not allow easy interpretation of the groups evolution over the years. Finally, it is worth noting that ICL prefers the simultaneous solution.

Table 16. Confusion table associated to the partition provided by the best independent clustering model retained by ICL

	Cluster 1	Cluster 2
Healthy	228	229
Bankruptcy	289	143

5. Conclusion

In this chapter, parametric transfer learning and parametric unsupervised transfer learning have been addressed for classification, regression or clustering problems when several samples are involved in the analysis. In each situation, the proposed transfer function belongs to a parametric family what allows to obtain an easy understanding of the functional link between populations. It corresponds also to a very flexible approach since (i) many constraints on the parametric link can be proposed from the most to the less restrictive ones and (ii) model selection allows to retain automatically the most appropriate constraint.

It is worth noting also that proposed strategies are all easy to implement by practitioners since they are finally quite close to standard methods. Shortly speaking, they correspond to particular simple, but meaningful, constraints on classical models.

Face to the huge amount of available data today and especially in a near future, transfer learning may also work as a powerful and generic data reduction tool. Indeed, it allows to identify links between populations and, as a consequence, it is a way to obtain equivalence classes for them.

Finally, some challenges have still to be addressed by this emerging field. For instance, it would be useful to extend the proposed methods to high dimensional data sets or to other classical techniques. In addition, it would interesting to weaken some assumptions as the exact variable concordance between variables, property which is currently required.

References

[1] D. M. Allen. The relationship between variable selection and data augmentation and a method for prediction. *Technometrics*, 16:125–127, **1974**.

[2] F. Beninel and C. Biernacki. ModÃ¨les d'extension de la rÃ©gression logistique. *Revue des Nouvelles Technologies de l'Information, Data Mining et apprentissage statistique : application en assurance, banque et marketing*, (A1):207–218, **2007**.

[3] C. Biernacki, F. Beninel, and V. Bretagnolle. A generalized discriminant rule when training population and test population differ on their descriptive parameters. *Biometrics*, 58(2):387–397, **2002**.

[4] C. Biernacki and G. Celeux. Assessing a mixture for clustering with the integrated completed likelihood. *IEEE Transactions on Pattern Analysis and Machine Intelligence*, 22:719–725, **2000**.

[5] C. Bouveyron and J. Jacques. Adaptive linear models for regression: improving prediction when population has changed. *Pattern Recognition Letters*, 31(14):2237–2247, **2010**.

[6] C. Bouveyron and J. Jacques. Adaptive mixtures of regressions: Improving predictive inference when population has changed. *Pub. IRMA Lille*, 70(VIII), **2010**.

[7] V. Bretagnolle. personnal communication. 2006.

[8] G. Celeux and G. Govaert. Clustering criteria for discrete data and latent class models. *Journal of Classification*, 8:157–176, **1991**.

[9] G. Celeux and G. Govaert. Parsimonious gaussian models in cluster analysis. *Pattern Recognition*, 28:781–793, **1995**.

[10] B. De Meyer, B. Roynette, P. Vallois, and M. Yor. On independent times and positions for Brownian motions. *Revista Matemática Iberoamericana*, 18(3):541–586, **2002**.

[11] A.P. Dempster, N.M. Laird, and D.B. Rubin. Maximum likelihood from incomplete data (with discussion). *Journal of the Royal Statistical Society. Series B*, 39:1–38, **1977**.

[12] P. Du Jardin and E. Séverin. Dynamic analysis of the business failure process: a study of bankruptcy trajectories. In *Portuguese Finance Network*, Ponte Delgada, Portugual, **2010**.

[13] B. S. Everitt. *An introduction to latent variable models*. Monographs on Statistics and Applied Probability. Chapman & Hall, London, 1984.

[14] C. Fraley and A. E. Raftery. How many clusters? Which clustering method? Answers via model-based cluster analysis. *Computer Journal*, 41:578–588, **1998**.

[15] M. Goldfeld and R.E. Quandt. A markov model for switching regressions. *Journal of Econometrics*, 1:3–16, **1973**.

[16] D. Hand. *Discriminant and Classification*. Wiley, New York, 1996.

[17] T. Hastie, R. Tibshirani, and J. Friedman. *The elements of statistical learning*. Springer Series in Statistics. Springer-Verlag, New York, 2009.

[18] C. Hennig. *Classification in the Information Age*. Springer-Verlag, Heidelberg, 1999.

[19] D.W. Hosmer and S. Lemeshow. *Applied logistic regression*. Wiley Series in Probability and Statistics. Wiley, 2000.

[20] M. Hurn, A. Justel, and C.P. Robert. Estimating mixtures of regressions. *Journal of Computational and Graphical Statistics*, 12(1):55–79, **2003**.

[21] J. Jacques and C. Biernacki. Extension of model-based classification for binary data when training and test populations differ. *Journal of Applied Statistics*, 37(5):749–766, **2010**.

[22] A. Lourme and C. Biernacki. Gaussian model-based classification when training and test population differ: Estimating jointly related parameters. In First joint meeting of the SociÃ©tÃ© Francophone de Classification and of the Classification and Data Analysis Group of SIS, 2008.

[23] A. Lourme and C. Biernacki. Simultaneous Gaussian Model-Based Clustering for Samples of Multiple Origins. *Computational Statistics, in press.*, **2012**.

[24] A. Lourme and C. Biernacki. Simultaneous t-model-based clustering for data differing over time period: Application for understanding companies financial health. *Case Studies in Business, Industry and Government Statistics (CSBIGS)*, 4(2), **2011**.

[25] G.J. McLachlan. *Discriminant analysis and statistical pattern recognition.* Wiley Series in Probability and Mathematical Statistics: Applied Probability and Statistics. John Wiley & Sons Inc., New York, 1992. , A Wiley-Interscience Publication.

[26] G.J. Mclachlan. *Discriminant Analysis and Statistical Pattern Recognition.* Wiley Series in Probability and Statistics. Wiley-Interscience, 2004.

[27] G.J. McLachlan and D. Peel. *Finite Mixture Models.* Wiley, New York, 2000.

[28] S.J. Pan and Q. Yang. A survey on transfer learning. *IEEE Transactions on knowledge and data engineering*, 22(10):1345–1359, **2010**.

[29] B. Ripley. *Pattern Recognition and Neural Network.* Cambridge University Press, Cambridge, 1995.

[30] K. Roeder and L. Wasserman. Practical Bayesian density estimation using mixtures of normals. *Journal of the American Statistical Association*, 92:894–902, **1997**.

[31] G. Schwarz. Estimating the dimension of a model. *The Annals of Statistics*, 6(2):461–464, **1978**.

[32] J.C. Thibault, V. Bretagnolle, and C. Rabouam. Cory's shearwater calonectris diomedea. *Birds of Western Paleartic Update*, 1:75–98, **1997**.

In: Knowledge Transfer: Practices, Types and Challenges
Editor: Dragan Ilic
ISBN: 978-1-62081-538-0

Chapter 6

PATTERNS OF KNOWLEDGE TRANSFER IN THE SPANISH BIOTECHNOLOGY INDUSTRY

***Beatriz Ortiz*[1], *Mario J. Donate*[2*] *and Fátima Guadamillas*[3]**

[1]University of Castilla-La Mancha, Faculty of Law and Social Sciences,
Department of Business Administration,
Cobertizo San Pedro Mártir s/n, Toledo, Spain

[2]University of Castilla-La Mancha, Faculty of Law and Social Sciences,
Department of Business Administration, Ronda de Toledo s/n, Ciudad Real, Spain

[3]University of Castilla-La Mancha, Faculty of Law and Social Sciences,
Department of Business Administration,
Cobertizo San Pedro Mártir s/n, Toledo, Spain

ABSTRACT

The biotechnology industry is characterized by a high intensity in knowledge creation and innovation. Biotechnology companies are constantly affected by knowledge flows so this industry is an interesting field to study knowledge transfer strategies. In this chapter we analyze the knowledge transfer strategies of three Spanish biotechnology companies, PharmaMar, Neocodex and Digna Biotech. With this aim an exploratory case study was carried out by the authors, which is based on the model of technological knowledge transfer developed by Bozeman (2000). The results of this study provide a comprehensive overview of the aspects that characterize different ways to understand a knowledge transfer strategy and the results that are obtained from its application.

1. INTRODUCTION

Nowadays the world lives a scientific and technological revolution that favors globalization and accelerates the development of new technologies. In this sense knowledge and technological innovation play a vital role in the industrial, economic and social

* Corresponding author: E-mail: mariojavier.donate@uclm.es

development of countries and their economies. In many businesses, innovation is achieved through the use of technology or technological knowledge (Escorsa and Valls, 2003), thus being the most important factor for competitive success (Shilling, 2008).

An innovation system could be defined as a complex set of relationships between various actors (companies, universities, public research institutes, etc.), that contribute to the development and dissemination of new technologies. They comprise a network where government policies can importantly influence the innovation process (Patel and Pavitt, 1994). In general terms, the efficiency of innovation systems is determined by their ability to transform knowledge into wealth. In this sense, technology transfer between the different system's actors is critical to achieving efficient performance (COTEC, 2010).

Knowledge transfer can be defined as the ability to move knowledge from one organizational unit into another, contributing positively to business performance (Argote and Ingram, 2000). Basically, knowledge transfer is based on the structuring and dissemination of knowledge within organizations, so that knowledge can be exploited effectively for productive purposes of the organization (Donate and Guadamillas, 2010).

In order to be innovative, companies should develop technological knowledge, which can be obtained from two complementary sources:

- Internal sources: research departments and technological development (R&D).
- External sources: collaboration with suppliers and external partners outside the company for technology acquisition when available, or purchases in the case of alliances are not possible to be established.

In this case (technology outside the company) technology transfer becomes one of the mechanism by which the company acquires resources or assets needed for innovation (González, 2011). The increasing complexity and multidisciplinarity of the resources needed to carry out technological innovations and the sharing of knowledge requires, in most cases, interaction and collaboration between different organizations with complementary resources (Arora and Gambardella, 1990). Sharing resources becomes absolutely necessary when the company is not able to internally develop all the knowledge required for their innovation process (Lundvall and Nielsen, 2003).

The biotechnology industry is nowadays regarded as one of the main drivers of technological change and it is crucial in accelerating the economic growth of many countries (Genome Spain, 2005). Life sciences are increasingly important in advanced societies, because these sciences are responsible for providing welfare to people, both in quantity and quality, along with key factors as food, energy and health care provision (Genome Spain, 2009). This industry is characterized by dynamism. It is an industry in which companies are constantly creating new knowledge and innovation. Biotech companies are continually managing knowledge flows, both internal and external (Decarolis and Deeds, 1999). The most valuable assets of biotechnology companies are their intangible research capabilities, which represent the potential to develop and distribute new drugs, different from traditional medicines provided by pharmaceutical companies. In addition, these companies are not only creating new products, but they are also seeking new research methods and new medical and diagnostic tools, very different from traditional pharmaceutical companies. This research capacity is derived from their knowledge, which must be continually nurtured and renewed (Grant, 2002). An appropriate context for examining flows of knowledge and its relationship to company performance is therefore a dynamic and innovative industry in terms of knowledge generation and exploitation, such as the biotechnology industry (Decarolis and Deeds, 1999).

In this research, the object of our study is knowledge transfer. The way in which transfer is developed it depends on the knowledge management strategy followed by companies. At the same time, each knowledge transfer strategy will have a different impact on company innovation performance (Donate and Guadamillas, 2010). Specifically, this paper suggests that the way patterns of knowledge transfer are developed by companies –i.e.., inter-company strategic guidance referred to the knowledge transfer– have an important influence on technological innovation outcomes of companies.

To justify this approach we rely on the fact that the acquisition of external knowledge is becoming one of the most important processes in knowledge management literatures (Donate and Guadamillas, 2010). Nowadays more companies, even the largest and most technologically self-sufficient, need to acquire knowledge beyond their boundaries (Cassiman and Veugelers, 2000). As noted above, in most cases companies are not able to make their own research or necessary work to implement product or process innovations, so access to partnership or acquisitions, can make this task easier (Diaz et al., 2001). Nevertheless the ability of companies to recognize the value of external knowledge it is not enough to make a technological innovation process succesful. In addition, companies have to be able to assimilate and apply knowledge for commercial purposes, issues that have become central for competitive success (Cohen and Levinthal, 1990) and are essential to correctly carry out knowledge transfer processes.

This fact is even more relevant in an industry such as Biotechnology, where large pharmaceutical companies, in order to face competition, try to improve their technological base by taking advantage of the innovation results of biotech companies, in order to continually launch new drugs to the market (Zeller, 2003).

The theoretical positioning of this paper is mainly based on the knowledge-based theory of the firm. This theory is based on the proposition that firms are bundles of unique resources and capabilities, where knowledge is the most strategically important (Grant, 1996). On the one hand, this approach makes a distinction between tacit knowledge, difficult to formalize and transmit, and explicit knowledge, which it can be codified and it is esily identifiable (Nonaka, 1991). The characteristics of knowledge influence the possibilities to be transferred, accumulated and exploited (Grant, 1996). It is thus important to take into account these knowledge features in order to effectively carry out knowledge transfer strategies.

Regarding methodology, we will analyse knowledge transfer strategies through the exhibition of prominent cases of three companies in the Biotechnology industry. Case study methodology is highly appropiate to deeply analyze descriptive and exploratory aspects in an empirical research (Yin, 1989 and 1993), and can generate theoretical propositions to be tested in future studies.

This chapter is structured as follows. Firstly we briefly explain the concept of technology transfer and discuss a general model based on Bozeman's (2000), through which we study knowledge transfer strategies. Next, we will show the case study of three biotech firms that have developed different knowledge transfer strategies to face competition in the industry and get innovation. Finally, conclusions will be drawn from the results obtained in the cases study.

2. External Transfer of Technological Knowledge

Technology transfer can be defined as the movement of technology and/or knowledge from one location to another, from a supplier (universities, research organizations, technology centers, firms...), to a recipient (usually firms) which acquires it for its exploitation in exchange for a compensation (González, 2011).

Another similar definition was depicted by Roessner (2000), who asserts that technology transfer is the movement of know-how, technological knowledge or technology from one organization to another; and COTEC (2003), also defines technology transfer as the transmission of intellectual capital and know-how among organizations with the purpose of their use in the creation and development of commercially viable products and services.

We can thus conclude that the transfer of technological knowledge is a process through which knowledge is transferred from a sending to a receiving unit.

Bozeman (2000) established a model with different elements that are part of the external process of technological knowledge transfer from a systemic point of view, trying to answer three main questions: (1) how external knowledge is acquired; (2) who acquired it; and (3) what environmental conditions surround the process of knowledge transfer.

The first of these issues, how external knowledge is acquired, is related to the technology transfer *agent*, the transfer *objectives* and the *means* by which the tecnological knowledge transfer is made. The analysis of these elements allows the identification of different patterns of technological knowledge transfer.

COTEC (2010) identifies the agents of technology transfer as those institutions or organizations that transfer the technology, and distinguishes the following types: suppliers of equipment, materials, components or software; clients; competitors or other kind of companies; consultants; commercial laboratories or private R&D institutes; universities or other higher education institutions; public research institutions; and finally, technology centers. A recent trend among companies is the use of cooperative agreements, especially in terms of R&D to acquire knowledge from the different agents previously pointed out (Veugelers, 1997; Fritseh and Lukas, 2001; Tether, 2002; Arora et al. 2001). Partnership is the development of knowledge through collaboration involving university relations, joint ventures, alliances and consortia of competitors, suppliers and customers (Fey and Birkinshaw, 2005).

Regarding the objectives and means for technological knowledge transfer, COTEC (2010) identifies the objectives as the transfer intention –i.e., to obtain knowledge and operational skills related to products, processes and production methods, machines and equipment, inputs, company organization methods and work. In accordance with Bozeman et al. (1995), the main aspects that are behind this objective would be the content, form, marketing opportunities, etc., of the object which is transferred.

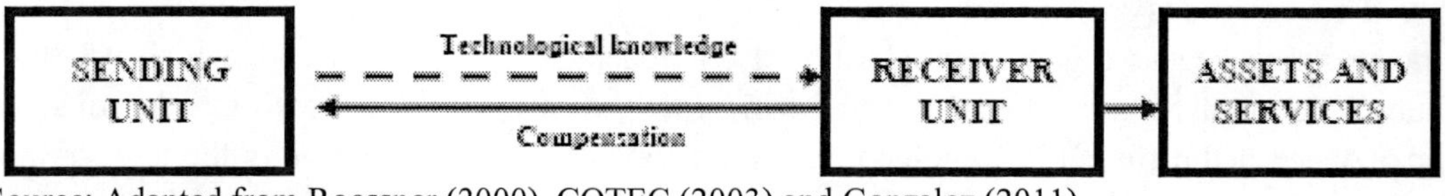

Source: Adapted from Roessner (2000), COTEC (2003) and Gonzalez (2011).

Figure 1. Concept of technological knowledge transfer.

Finally, Carayol (2003) defines the means for transfer as the instrument, formal or informal, by which the knowledge and/or technology is transferred, that can be classified as: tacit knowledge transfer, which is informally made through personal exchange of information, workshops, fairs, etc...; explicity transfer, made through formal tools that can be contractual or not, such as patents, licensing, contract research, training, staff exchanges, etc...; and embedded transfer, referred to knowledge or technology that can be appropiated through the acquisition of machinery, equipment or other kind of devices (COTEC, 2010).

The second issue addressed by Bozeman (2000) to establish the model of technology transfer is based on determining who purchase the technology, establishing their characteristics in terms of absorption capacity, resources, strategies, location, etc. For instance, companies, agencies, consumers, governments or public institutions, etc. (Harmon et al., 1997). The analysis of the recipient of the technological knowledge allows the elaboration of different taxonomies, according the above features, which it also promotes technology transfer to a greater or a lesser degree. The third and final question that tries to answer the transfer model of Bozeman (2000) refers to those factors (market or otherwise) related to the need of the transferred object within the socio-cultural environment (technology/knowledge price, substitutability, relationship with the technology/knowledge currently in use, grants, captive markets, etc..) and it determines the external conditions that make agents with similar characteristics to behave in a differentiated way (COTEC, 2010).

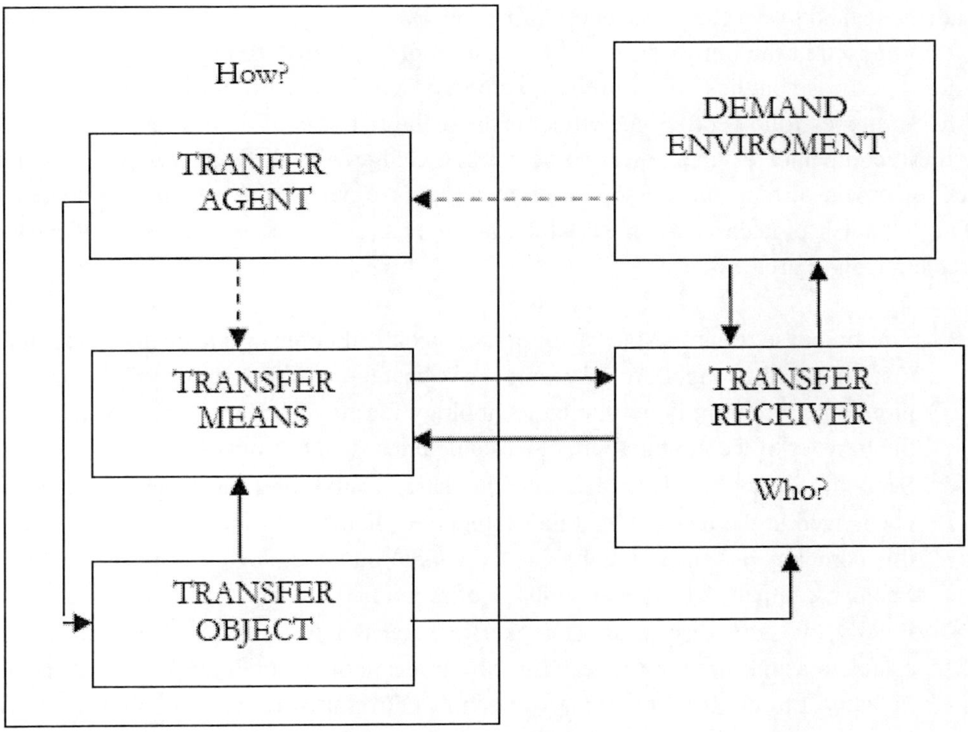

Source: Adapted from Bozeman (2000).

Figure 2. Transfer Model of Technological Knowledge.

The environment analysis allows the assessment of the supportive elements and obstacles and limits to innovation that could be present in the environment in which any organization operates. This model represents, among other benefits, a complete overview of the issues that comprehensively characterize a representation of technology and knowledge transfer. It can also be very useful in determining different technological patterns that characterize a particular industry or country, and it could be use to analyze the influence of environmental conditions on the choice of patterns for each type of agent. For this reason, this model has been used in this research as the basis of our analysis, since in our view this model could be useful to study knowledge transfer strategies in the Spanish biotech industry.

3. Case Study Analysis

Case studies could be defined as a research method that is characterized by the study of processes within real contexts using multiple sources of evidence, with the aim to explain observed phenomena as a whole and taking into account their complexity.

It allows researchers to face questions about the "how" and "why" a phenomenom occur (Yin, 1989; 1993). Moreover, it facilitates the use of multiple methods of data collection, and allows researchers to a deeper examination of the phenomenon under study.Case study methodology is also an adequate way to explore research issues for which the existing theory is inadequate, and to develop new theory (Yin, 1993).

As proposed in the introduction section, and in order to analyse technological knowledge transfer, three case studies will allow the authors to check for different types of knowledge transfer strategies followed by biotech companies, the richness of their knowledge flows and how these companies exchange technological knowledge with different agents associated to the development of their businesses. In order to achieve our purpose we have selected three cases of Spanish biotech companies, which are a clear reference within their industry. The chosen companies are:

- The first case, PharmaMar, is a biopharmaceutical company dedicated to explore the marine world in the search for innovative therapies. This company has conducted a pioneering program in marine biotechnology for the discovery of new drugs in which the transfer of technology with other companies is an essential aspect.
- Secondly we will analyse the Neocodex case, a small biotechnology company that it is engaged in the research and development of human genetics. Despite its small size this company has made great achievements in biotechnology, such as being the first Spanish company owning a data-bank of around 20,000 DNA samples.
- Finally, we will discuss the Digna Biotech case, a company that was created to establish a link between research in the biotechnology field and the pharmaceutical industry. In only 9 years Digna Biotech has developed a solid and ambitious project for basic and applied research in biomedicine.

2.1. Pharmamar: Pharmacy at Sea

3.1.1. Company Description

PharmaMar, S.A. was created in 1986 and is part of a group of companies comprising the Zeltia Group, founded more than 60 years ago. Since its foundation in 1939, Zeltia has always been involved in the chemical-pharmaceutical industry.

PharmaMar, with over 250 employees, is among the leading Spanish pharmaceutical companies that invest more in research, development and innovation. During its first 20 years of development, it spent more than 450 million € in R&D&i. PharmaMar's corporate strategy is based on discovering, developing and commercializing products of marine origin applied for medical treatments against cancer.

3.1.2. Knowledge Transfer Model

With regard to the way that PharmaMar manages knowledge flows, firtly it is interesting to analyse its role as a recipient agent of technological knowledge. The way PharmaMar acquires knowledge is mainly based on establishing partnerships with various actors, from suppliers of marine compounds to Governments, Universities, hospitals and scientific institutions, with the aim of discovering new drugs of marine origin. Specifically, PharmaMar has established an extensive network worldwide, comprising more than 60 marine biology centers, chemistry and cancer biology researchers, in order to expand the investigation into its extensive collection of potentially active agents. This network includes centers of biochemistry and marine biology, which has been provided access to marine samples (micro and macro), as well as basic science researchers and world class clinics. Similarly, it has worked with local governments and institutions to explore local biodiversity and establish joint discovery programs of new anti-cancer compounds obtained from the sea. It is also important for the company to maintain an ongoing commitment to establish partnerships in the clinical development context and determine the molecular basis of action mechanisms of its anti-cancer compounds. Near to 100 Universities, hospitals, and scientific institutions around the world in the field of clinical development work together with PharmaMar.

Moreover, the means by which this technological knowledge transfer occurs have both tacit and informal character, and explicit and formal as well. Tacit knowledge transfer occurs, particularly, through the PharmaMar participation in numerous scientific meetings[3]. Patents are the main instrument used by PharmaMar to transfer knowledge. PharmaMar has a portfolio consisting of more than 1,800 patents, where about 1,300 are granted patents, and over 500 patent applications are still pending of approval. Such records are gathered in 97 patent families, each of which it protects a given invention. It is noteworthy to point out that

[3] For example, PharmaMar has participated in congresses both national (II Biotechnology and Business Congress in Barcelona, Pamplona BioSpain, both held in 2010, among others) and international (52 Annual Meeting of the American Society of Hematology (ASH) in 2010, the first forum of marine Biotechnology of the Academy of Sciences New York Oncology Congress or the American Society of Clinical Oncology (ASCO) held in 2011, among others). Moreover it regularly participates in trade fairs, such as Fair Ibero-American Science, Technology and Innovation (Empírika) and Workshops as XVIII workshop on "Advances in molecular biology". These are just some examples of the many scientific meetings in which PharmaMar participates (Corporate Social Responsibility Report Zeltia Group, 2010), in which, as noted above, there is an intensive exchange of tacit and informal knowledge.

one third of all patents and scientific publications on marine-derived anti-cancer drugs are the result of the internal research carried out by PharmaMar.

In order to finish the depiction of the transfer model through which PharmaMar acquires knowledge, we will identify areas that characterize the environment in which such transfer occurs. The biotechnology sector in Spain is an emerging industry with a fragmented market, whose financial structure has to support large investments without, in many cases, finishing in product commercialization. Moreover, most of the R&D projects are long-term oriented, which requires a large investment for development that introduces risks and uncertainty into the final results to obtain (Genome Spain, 2005).

In the task of mitigating these problems and achieving sucess in R&D, PharmaMar has been supported by public institutions in Spain. For example, in 2009 the company has obtained funding from the Center for Industrial Technology Development (CDTI). PharmaMar has also obtained funds from the R&D&i Technology Parks Program of the Ministry of Science and Innovation. Finally, funds for other projects were approved in 2009, such as the Business Innovation Program (PIE), Madrid Development Institute, and the Biotechnology and Biopharmaceutical Program of the Department of Economics, Statistics and Technological Innovation in the Community of Madrid, Spain.

From the strategy followed by PharmaMar we also find that this firm does not only play the role of technological knowledge recipient, but it also generates and transfers knowledge to other agents. For example, PharmaMar has established a licensing policy for the marketing of its product outside Europe, except in the case of the commercialization of compounds that show activity in different therapeutic oncology areas, whose licenses are granted worldwide. Moreover, as mentioned above, PharmaMar has established research contracts with centers in biochemistry and marine biology, which have provided access to its marine samples porfolio, as well as basic science researchers and clinics around the world.

Similarly, it is interesting to note the role of training provided by PharmaMar to the scientific community as a mechanism of knowledge transfer. PharmaMar supports the training of young scientists, by means of agreements with Spanish and foreign Universities, and it relies on the value of partnerships and transfer of technical knowledge as a tool to promote science and research for the future Society welfare. It has also developed agreements and grants with several national and international Universities and invests an important amount of financial resources in training and development of its employees. Overall, a range of agents acquires the knowledge produced and transferred by PharmaMar. On the one hand, a number of companies or institutions buy its licenses, usually large pharmaceutical corporations such as the Japanese company Taiho Pharmaceutical, which acquired the Yondelis license – leading cancer drug that PharmaMar launched in 2007– or the products of Johnson and Johnson U.S. subsidiary Ortho Biothech, with which PharmaMar maintains a licensing agreement for the same product since 2001. On the other hand, local communities and educational institutions (research institutes, universities, etc.) also acquire PharmaMar technical knowledge. These organisations find advantages from using the archive of samples of PharmaMar, which it brings together more than 95,000 marine samples from the highest biodiversity areas in the world. PharmaMar shares detailed reports of the marine ecosystems thus providing a new understanding or the concept of the sea ecosystem. Finally, the researchers and scientists who work or collaborate with PharmaMar, receive flows of technical knowledge developed within the company, becoming thus recipients of the firm's technology.

3.1.3. Conclusion: Pharmamar's Model of Technological Knowledge Transfer

The knowledge transfer strategy carried out by PahrmaMar can be analyzed from two points of view since PharmaMar is both recipient and provider of technological knowledge. The knowledge transfer model can be thus considered from two different perspectives, as shown in Figure 3.

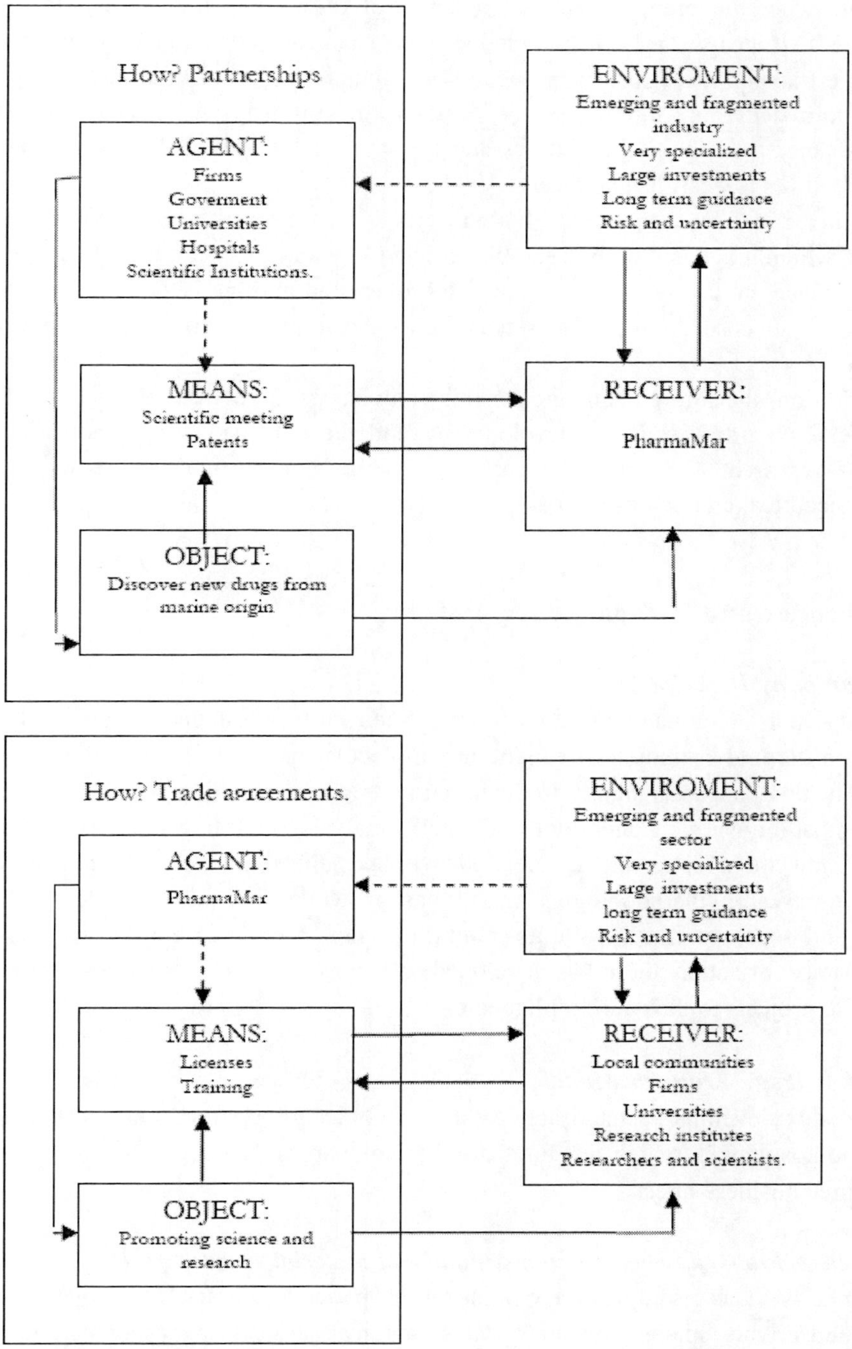

Source: Adapted from Bozeman (2000).

Figure 3. PharmaMar's model of technological knowledge transfer.

On the one hand, PharmaMar acquires not only technological knowledge from other companies, governmental and scientific institutions with the aim of discovering new drugs, but it also transfers its knowledge to these agents through licensing or training with the objective of promoting science and research.

PharmaMar therefore transfers technological knowledge by means both of cooperation agreements where the company acts as a receiver of knowledge, and commercial agreements, in which it assumes the role of knowledge provider. From our point of view PharmaMar's knowledge transfer strategy is very successful, since in this kind of environment where the flows of knowledge are intense and continuous, the company performance depends on the firm's capacity to manage these flows and accumulate the knowledge they generate better than competitors (Decarolis and Deeds, 1999).

This fact is reflected in recent PharmaMar's successes, such as the approval of the drug Yondelis, which it is being used in the EU for the treatment of sarcoma, and has recently been commercialised in the U.S. and Japan. Moreover PharmaMar is having talks with other companies to license Aplidin, the second most developed treatment in the world against cancer.

In addition, the future challenge for this company is the achievement of similar success for new compounds in clinical development, and the expansion of its potential to earlier stages of research. For all these reasons, PharmaMar is one of the most promising biopharmaceutical companies in Spain.

3.2. Neocodex and its Genetic Analysis

3.2.1. Company Description

Neocodex is a company based on Seville, Spain. It was founded in 2002 and its mission is focus on the understanding of genetic and molecular basis of common diseases in human beings. The company was mainly founded with the aim of combining the use of biomaterials with the most innovative technologies of genetic analysis, providing solutions to discover and focus on new therapeutic targets. Neocodex is specialized in the development and use of innovative research methodologies and it has grown to become a leader in biomedical research and development. Despite its small dimension, around 25 employees, Neocodex has large capacity for action and it has developed an extensive range of services, from the design of scientifc projects to their full implementation.

3.2.2. Knowledge Transfer Model

Neocodex develops its main activity as a knowledge supplier, since it is a provider of services to hospitals, research institutes or other companies. Neocodex organizes its activities around three business lines:

1) *DNA Biobank, which contains biological material from more than 20,000 different people.* These samples are obtained from patients' extractions of twenty five public and private Spanish hospitals, whose medical services are responsible for collecting samples without receiving any benefit in return, except the rights of royalty on patents that Neocodex develops. In addition, Neocodex offers its expertise to other

developing biobanks that receive direct advice from the company on how to manage the process. For example, the Alzheimer Foundation from Murcia (Spain) commissioned Neocodex a neuroprotection project to create the largest genetic database on Alzheimer in Spain.

2) *DNA scanning technology*. The Neocodex's technology platform of multiple reading is oriented to the massive reading of DNA, which it allows scientists to perform genetic analyses very quickly. With this service Hospitals such as the Virgen Macarena in Seville has discovered two new genes involved in the arising of multiple sclerosis. Moreover, since 2007, the Spanish company Corporación Dermoestética has got an agreement with Neocodex through which offers its customers the possibility of a detailed study of DNA. This study shows, for instance, their predisposition to suffer from obesity, heart risks and other diseases such as cancer or Alzheimer.
3) *Bioinformatics*. Neocodex's research is aimed at designing new mathematical tools for the development and analysis of high-density genetic panels, derived from whole genome scans. For example, it has patented the HFCC system, which it has been developed to meet the growing needs of pharmacogenomics and genetic research, where the conventional interpretation of genetic data is insufficient. Projects such as neuroprotection, previously mentioned, it is based on the use of this tool in order to isolate and characterize the molecular pathways involved in common neurodegenerative diseases that are more prevalent among the Spanish population, such as Alzheimer.

In addition to these contractual arrangements, Neocodex has established numerous partnerships with universities and public research organizations, developing programs of joint research, both national, such as PARKS and PROFIT projects, and European, such as GENEDISRUPT. It is also a member of several associations such as the Technological Corporation of Andalusia, the ASEBIO Bioenterprises Association, or the ONCOLOGICA business consortium, for the research and development of new cancer treatments. Overall, the aim of these agreements is the creation of value through the discovery and development of pre-products or pro-drugs to nurtur standardized processes for developing new drugs and discovering the genetic and molecular basis of the most common diseases in human beings. The company philosophy is to develop these pre-products, and complete pre-clinical stages of these. In so doing they try to obtain intellectual property to develop diagnosis and treatments for diseases under study. Regarding the way by which the knowledge transfer occurs, Neocodex participates in numerous conferences, seminars and workshops[4] that are used by the firm to capture explicit and tacit knowledge, along with research contracts, patents, training and personnel exchanges.

Neocodex has registered six patents on medical issues as diverse as cardiovascular treatments, osteoporosis processes or menopause. The company pays royalties to the hospitals that help to develop the patents, conducts training by participating in the Master in Human

[4] During the year 2011 Neocodex participated in the VII Congress Multidisciplinary Head and Neck Cancer, hosted by the Polytechnic University of Cartagena, or the Third Conference on Bioethics, organized by UCAM. Other scientific meetings in which it has participated are Neocodex eg BioContad Québec 2008, held in Canada, or the organization of the International Workshop "Genome wide scans for disease susceptibility," both events held during 2008.

Genetics of the Seville University, and bring its own staff to those companies that demand its services, when required.

Among the various means for transferring technical knowledge that Neocodex uses, we also find its own subsidiary in the U.S., and it is planning to expand its activitiesto other countries such as Japan and Iran. Moreover, despite its recent foundation (9 years), it has already generated a start-up, Neocodex Reprofiling, created with the aim of finding non-patented drug applications for medicines that have already been developed, in order to decrease expenses by taking advantages from the Neocodex's accumulated knowledge base.

The last issue of the model proposed by Bozeman (2000) is related to the management of the company's environment. As in the previous case (PharmaMar), the market is fragmented, and there is great uncertainty for every developed product.

Neocodex has an important advantage in terms of funds since it has financial resources from venture capital firms, as well as grants and loans from the Spanish Goverment. In so doing the company has secured the acquisition of resources to finance new projects. Neocodex developed in its early years a partnership with a high added-value investor, which not only contributed to the firm with monetary resources, but it got to related Neocodex to other investors and offered its expertise in politics, management or finance fields.

In turn, this expertise has been instrumental for the Neocodex development, and although it has undergone several capital increases that have significantly diluted the participation of its founding partners, the company has got resources in order to fluently evolve in its projects.

3.2.3. Conclusion: Neocodex's Model of Technological Knowledge Transfer

Figure 4 shows that the Neocodex's model of technological knowledge transfer is based primarily on its role as a supplier of knowledge. Neocodex knowledge is commercialized and transmitted to hospitals, scientific and research institutes or other biotechnology companies. The content of that knowledge is based on giving an understanding of the genetic and molecular basis of common diseases in human beings and creating business value through the discovery and development of pre-products encoded in intellectual property instruments (patents).

The means by which this transfer produces are formal (royalties, training and exchange of staff), informal (scientific meetings) and incorporated (creation of subsidiaries and the start-up Neocodex Reprofiling).

The environment in which Neocodex develops its activity has the same characteristics than any other biotechnology company in Spain, requiring large investments given its long-term orientation and uncertainty.

In this sense, a peculiarity for Neocodex has been the opportunity to have a major venture capital investor since its early years, a situation that is not very common in the Spanish biotechnology industry.

From our viewpoint the posibility to access to financial resources has been one of the most influential factors for the success of the Neocodex's knowledge transfer strategy, through which it has got a number of achievements, such as the building of the largest DNA data-bank in Spain, six patents and the publication of more than 50 scientific articles, a profit of more than half a million euros in just over 6 years since its foundation, or a stable flow of incomes that makes Neocodex to become quite independent of public borrowing.

In the near future the company is also planning to grow internationally and build the group Neocodex, a biotechnology holding company focused on technology transfer, bioinformatics and genetic diagnosis.

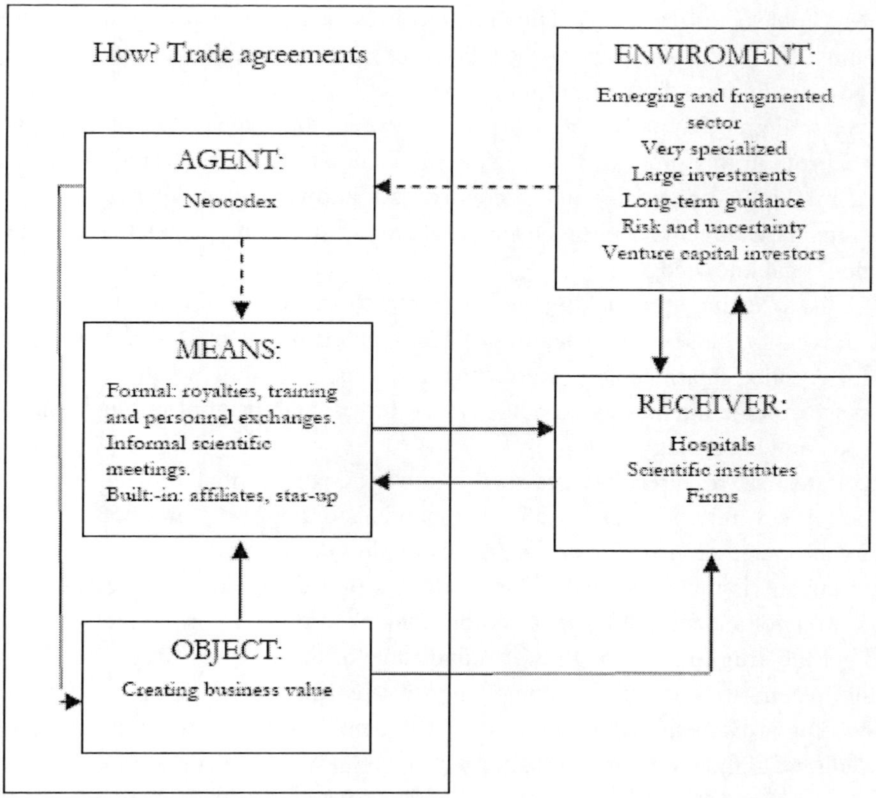

Source: Adapted from Bozeman (2000).

Figure 4. Neocodex's model of technological knowledge transfer.

3.3. Digna Biotech: Links between Science and Industry

3.3.1. Company Description

Digna Biotech is a biotechnology company focused on the development and exploitation of research products that are generated in the Centre for Applied Medical Research (CIMA) in Pamplona, Spain. It was founded on February 2003, and it has another work center operating in Madrid, Spain. The company emerged from the joint venture of CIMA, which is owned by the Foundation for Applied Medical Research (FIMA). Its main objective is the search for commercial applications of CIMA patents, one of the institutions that posseses a largest number of protected biotechnological inventions in Spain. Since its foundation, the company has got a large group of people with scientific and managerial experience in the field of the biomedical research. Its staff consists of 20 employees and it also receives external advice from various service companies in the areas of human resource management, accounting and law.

3.3.2. Knowledge Transfer Model

Digna Biotech is an example of the role undertaken by some recently established biotechnology companies, whose transformation process allows the mobilization and productive use of knowledge that is generated in research centers for the use of larger companies (Fontes, 2001; 2003). Digna Biotech is currently working to bridge the gap between the knowledge generated by the CIMA researchers and its commercialization, so this knowledge can be transformed into new products manufactured by the pharmaceutical industry. In so doing, Digna becomes the link between both types of institutions, and it thus plays a dual role in this process; firstly, as a knowledge recipient in terms of patents that are developed by the own company; and secondly, as a knowledge supplier, since the company transfers this knowledge through licensing to pharmaceutical companies that are interested in this technological knowledge.

CIMA is a leading private biomedical research center in Spain. It is located at the Navarra University, close to the Faculties of Medicine, Biology and Pharmacy, and the CIFA (Center for Applied Pharmacology Research), and aims at finding solutions to the first stage of diseases in four clinical areas: oncology, cardiovascular pathophysiology, neuroscience, gene therapy and hepatology.

This branch of research has drawn a number of patents that protects the commercial exploitation of several potentially useful therapeutic and diagnostic products. For this reason, Digna Biotech was established to commercially exploit these patents.

The company is thus responsible for producing molecules or compounds that the CIMA discovers, in amounts enough to be tested on humans in order to prove their effectivity. The aim is to get the drug to go through the second stage of the research (as required by law) and obtain the patent to license the compound to any interested pharmaceutical company. Nowadays, Digna Biotech has got more than 40 patents, of which the company has selected those based on a higher commercial viability to move through the commercialization process.

On the other hand, and in order to achieving a sustainable development of its products, Digna Bioctech has developed several partnerships with other companies. For example, it has recently established a cooperation agreement with the French firm *Flamel Technologies*, which will carry out the design and manufacturing of certain Digna products.

Moreover, Digna Biotech does not only develop patented products for the CIMA, but it also develops products patented by other companies. In 2009, Digna Biotech established an alliance with the companies *Biotecnol* and *Genentech*. This alliance granted Digna and Biotecnol an exclusive right over one of the patents of Genentech that permits both companies to develop new products for the treatment of liver diseases.

With regard to the achievement of its objective of being a provider of technological patented knowledge, Digna has got licence agreements for seven patents since the company was created, which have allowed it to start to work on the development of new products from the beginning of the value-chain process. For instance, some of these agreements through licensing are: a product for the Ferrer pharmaceutical group; two pharmaceutical products for ISDIN (a specialized laboratory in dermatology); and a preferencial agreement with Amsterdam Molecular Therapeutics (AMT).

In exchange for these agreements Digna Biotech receives financial returns and royalties. Another way by which Digna Biotech carries out knowledge transfer to other companies is through its participation at numerous scientific meetings, such as BioSpain 2010, or the "cooperation days" between pharmaceutical and biotechnology companies in the area of

Neurosciences, organized by Farmaindustria to facilitate collaboration in the development of new drugs.

Regarding environmental issues in knowledge transfer (Bozeman, 2000), Digna Biotech has received support since its foundation by an investment group, formed by some of the major Spanish companies, such as BBVA and the Corte Inglés, as well as by several foundations, including the Foundation for Applied Medical Research (FIMA) and the Navarra University Foundation (FUNA), along with savings banks such as Caja Rural de Navarra and Caixa Galicia.

Overall, Digna constitutes a joint venture formed by 15 partners. Moreover, Digna Biotech has received significant public financial support, such as CDTI credits and grants awarded by the Navarra regional Government. This financial support along with the incomes obtained from licensing has made possible the development of a large number of patents produced by the CIMA and their consequent development by Digna Biotech.

3.3.3. Conclusion: Digna Biotech's Model of Technological Knowledge Transfer

By analyzing the Digna Biotech's model of technological knowledge transfer, we can assert that the most important feature of its technological knowledge transfer strategy is based on its dual role as an agent receiving and transmitting knowledge as reflected in Figure 5.

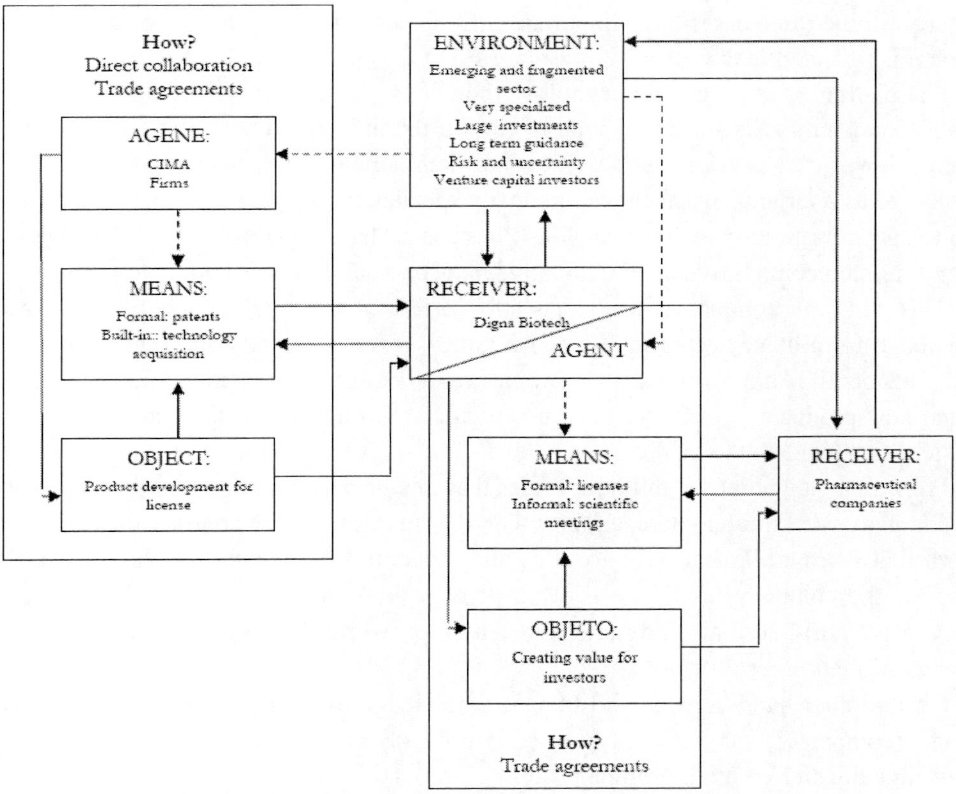

Source: Adapted from Bozeman (2000).

Figure 5. Digna Biotech's model of technological knowledge transfer.

As a recipient agent, Digna Biotech acquires knowledge from the CIMA, which is responsible for generating patentable research products in the first stage of the research. In this sense the patent is the instrument through which the company acquires knowledge by means of a formal transfer of technological knowledge.

On the other side, Digna Biotech conducts a number of trade agreements with other companies to outsource product manufacturing. The purpose is to develop products in early stages of the research, being possible to license patents to pharmaceutical companies. The license is thus the formal mechanism used by Digna to transfer knowledge with the objective to generate added value to its investors.

CONCLUSION

Throughout this chapter we have tried to analyze knowledge transfer in three Spanish biotech companies, PharmaMar, Neocodex and Digna Biotech. To fulfill this purpose, we have based the analysis on the model of technological knowledge transfer proposed by Bozeman (2000), which establishes different technological patterns that characterize a particular industry or country. We have also analyed the influence that enviromental conditions has on the behavioral patterns followed by knowledge transfer agents.

Overall the three cases have important differences that affect their knowledge strategies, which it is reflected in table 1.

PharmaMar is a large biotechnology company, subsidiary of a highly consolidated corporation (Zeltia, S.A). It has a long history in the industry and a solid financial structure, which allows it to develop its activities and commercialize its own products. It could be considered as a large pharmaceutical company specialized in marine biotechnology products. Due to specialization, companies such as PharmaMar have a permanent need for research in order to remain competitive in an innovative industry such as biotechnology.

This kind of companies needs also to internally develop technology, and acquires knowledge from other agents such as universities, research centers and other firms. In most cases, this combination of internal development and external acquisition allows companies to launch new products in order to be commercialized through licensing, and in so doing, they transfer knowledge to the market.

From this viewpoint we might consider that this behavior pattern could be developed by any company with similar characteristics than PharmaMar. On the contrary the case study has shown that PharmaMar not only acquires and transfers knowledge with the aim of creating value for the company (as Digna Biotech or Neocodex make when they develop the same behavior pattern) but to also promote research, improve people welfare, train employees, and share investigation results.

On the other hand, agents who transfer knowledge to PharmaMar are the same type of agents (companies, governments, scientific institutions and universities) that obtain knowledge transferred by the company.

This may be motivated by the extensive network of relationships that this company has developed over the years, which allows it to promote research among the network that will provide technological knowledge to obtain new drugs. We can thus conclude that there is a reciprocal relationship of the flows of technological knowledge between PharmaMar and the rest of the network agents.

Unlike PharmaMar, Digna Biotech and Neocodex are small start-ups that have achieved many accomplishments in a short period of time, primarily because they have received significant venture capital investments.

Table 1. Cases comparison

	PharmaMar		Neocodex	Digna Biotech	
Foundation year	1986		2002	2003	
Employees	Over 250		Less than 25	Less than 25	
Main knowledge transfer pattern	Recipient	Supplier	Supplier	Recipient	Supplier
Alliances	Collaborations	Trade	Trade	Collaboration s and Trade	Trade
Transmitter/ Recipient	Firms Goverment Universities Hospitals Scientific Institutions	Local communities Firms Universities Research institutes Researchers and scientists	Firms, Research institutions Hospitals	CIMA Firms	Pharmace utical firms
Object	Drug discovery	Promoting research	Creating business value	Development licensed products	Creating business value
Means	Formal and informal	Formal	Formal, informal and built-in	Formal and built-in	Formal and informal
External financial dependence	Low		High	High	

Source: Authors.

Such small companies usually require the cooperation of large firms to develop and commercialize their products, since they do not have financial and organizational resources to develop innovations on their own. In general, these small biotech companies play the role of technological knowledge providers of larger companies, for instance, through the provision of services such as R&D outsourcing –the Neocodex case– or licensing their patented products. This fact is reflected in the behavior pattern of companies such as Digna and Neocodex. We have also observed that Digna Biotech has played an intermediate role between a biotech research institute, CIMA, and large pharmaceutical companies, acquaring and transferring technological knowledge at the same time.

An important difference has been found in relation to the way the knowledge transfer process ocurrs for the three companies. When we observe their role as recipients of technological knowledge, PharmaMar and Digna Biotech choose patents as the main instrument for the formal transfer, while PharmaMar use informal means such as scientific meetings, and Digna Biotech also acquires technology to external firms when it outsources the manufacturing function of its value chain. On the other hand we observe the use of formal means to transfer knowledge, such as licensing and training, when we consider the role of the three firms as knowledge providers. In this point we have to highlight the informal means of knowledge transfer used by Digna Biotech and Neocodex, such as their participation in scientific meetings.

Overall, Neocodex is the company that uses more instruments to transfer knowledge. In our opinion, this fact may be motivated by the distinctive characteristics of this firm as a technological knowledge provider instead of a recipient, which it is found to be present to a greater extent in PharmaMar and Digna Biotech.

Although this study is exploratory and we are aware that the results have to be confirmed in subsequent studies, we have importantly showed three cases of Spanish firms with different patterns of knowledge transfer. These patterns do not only derive from organizational characteristics and environmental elements, although the access to financial resources is a key issue in this industry, as we have stressed throughout this chapter. Moreover, we have found for the three cases that, even in a company such as Neocodex, where it appears that knowledge transfer is produced in a one-way direction, knowledge flows do not follow a single path. Conversely, in this complex and dynamic industry knowledge exchanges occur quickly and continously, and knowledge flows are produced in both directions. Surely the success for firms in this industry in the near future will depend on the velocity and quality of knowledge transfer, along with their capacity to assimilate, accumulate and exploit knowledge for getting technological innovation and competitive advantages.

REFERENCES

Alavi, M. and Leidner, D. (2001), "Knowledge Management and Knowledge Management Systems: Conceptual Foundations and Research Issues", *MIS Quarterly*, 25 (1): 107-136.

Argote L. and Ingram P. (2000), "Knowledge transfer: a basis for competitive advantage in firms", *Organizational Behaviour and Human Decision Processes*, 82: 150-169.

Arora, A. and Gambardella, A (1990); "Complementarity and External Linkages: The Strategies of the Large Firms in Biotechnology", *The Journal of Industrial Economics*, 38(4): 361-379.

Arora, A., Fosfuri, A. and Gambardella, A. (2001), *Markets for Technology: Economics of Innovation and Corporate Strategy*, MIT Press, Cambridge, MA.

Bozeman, B. (2000), "Technology transfer and public policy: a review of research and theory", *Research Policy*, 29: 627-655.

Bozeman, B., Papadakis, M. and Coker, K. (1995), "Industry perspectives on commercial interactions with federal laboratories: does the cooperative technology paradigm really work?", *National Science Foundation. Research on Science and Technology Program*, January.

Carayol, N. (2003), "Objectives, agreements and matching in science-industry collaborations: reassembling the pieces of the puzzle", *Research Policy,* 32(6): 887-908.

Cassiman, B. and Veugelers, R. (2000), "External Technology Sources: Embodied or Disembodied Technology Acquisition", University Pompeu Fabra, *Economics and Business Working Paper*, No. 444.

Cohen, W.M. and Levinthal, D.A. (1990), "Absorptive Capacity: A New Perspective on Learning and Innovation", *Administrative Science Quarterly*, Special Issue: Technology, Organizations, and Innovation, 35(1): 128-152.

COTEC (2003), *New mechanisms of technology transfer*, COTEC Foundation for Technological Innovation, Madrid.

COTEC, (2010), Technology transfer in Spanish companies: *patterns identification according PITEC panel*. Madrid.

Decarolis, D.M. and Deeds, D.L. (1999), "The impact of stocks and flows of Organizational Knowledge on Firm Performance: an empirical investigation of the biotechnology industry", *Strategic Management Journal,* 20: 953-968.

Diaz, V., Muñoz, E. and J. Espinosa (2001), *"The biotechnology company in Spain: a first map of an innovative sector,"* Working Paper 01-01. Comparative Policies Unit (CSIC).

Donate, M.J. y Guadamillas, F. (2010), "The Effect of Organizational Culture on Knowledge Management Practices and Innovation", *Knowledge and Process Management*, 17(2): 82-94.

Escorsa, P. and Valls, J. (2003), *Technology and Innovation in the company*, UPC Editions, Barcelona.

Fey, C. y Birkinshaw, J. (2005), "External Sources of Knowledge, Governance Mode, and R&D Performance", *Journal of Management*, 31(4): 597-621.

Fontes, M. (2001), "The process of transformation of scientific and technological knowledge into economic value as conducted by academic spin-offs", *Proceedings of the R&D Management Conference*, 6-7 September 2001, Dublin: NITM, 159- 167.

Fontes, M. (2003), "Distant Networking: The Knowledge Acquisition Strategies of "out-cluster" Biotechnology Firms", *Proceedings of DRUID Summer Conference* , 12-14 June 2003, Copenhaguen.

Fritsch, M. y Lukas, R.. (2001), "Who cooperate on R&D?", *Research Policy,* 30: 297-312.

Genome Spain, (2005), Spanish Biotechnology: economic impact, trends and prospects, Madrid.

Genome Spain, (2009), Relevance of Biotechnology in Spain 2009, Madrid.Gonzalez, J. (2011), Handbook of technology and knowledge transfer, *Technology and Knowledge Transfer Institute*. www.thetransferinstitute.com/publications.

Grant, R.M. (1996), "Toward a knowledge Based Theory of the firm", *Strategic Management Journal*, 17(1): 109-122.

Grant, R.M. (2002), *Contemporary Strategy Analysis. Concepts, Techniques and Applications* (4th ed). Blackwell Publishers: Boston: MA.

Harmon, B., Ardishvili, A., Cardozo, R.., Elder, T., Leuthold, J., Parshall, J., Raghian, M. and Smith, M. (1997), "Mapping the university technology transfer process", *Journal of Business Venturing,* 12(6): 423-434.

Nielsen P. adnd Lundvall, B. (2003), "Innovation, Learning Organizations and Industrial Relations", *DRUID Working Paper 03-07.*

Patel, P. and Pavitt, K. (1994): "The Nature and Economic Importance of National Innovation Systems", *Science Technology Industry Review*, OCDE, 14: 343-373.

Quintana, C. and Benavides C.A. (2004), *"National systems of biotechnology innovation. An international comparison ",* Revista Asturiana de Economía, 30: 87-114.

Roessner; J.D. (2000), "Technology transfer" en Hill. C. (Ed.) *Science and Technology policy in te U.S. A time of Change.* Longman:London.

Schilling, M.A. (2008), *Strategic Management of technological innovation*, McGraw-Hill Irwin, Boston.

Spender J.C. and Grant R.M. (1996), "Knowledge and the firm: overview", *Strategic Management Journal*, 17 (Winter Special Issue), pp. 5-9.

Tether, B. (2002), "Who cooperates for innovation, and why: an empirical analysis", *Research Policy*, 31: 947-967.

Veugelers, R.. (1997), "Internal R&D expenditures and external technology sourcing", *Research Policy*, 26: 303–315.

Yin, R. K. (1989), *Case Study Research. Design and Methods*, Newbury Park, CA: Sage.

Yin, R. K. (1993), *Applications of Case Study Research*, Newbury Park, CA: Sage.

Zeller, C. (2003); "Restructuring Knowledge Acquisition and Production in the Pharmaceutical and Biotech Industries", en V. LoandE. Schamp (eds) *Knowledge –The Spatial Dimension*, Münster: Lit-Verlag.

In: Knowledge Transfer: Practices, Types and Challenges
Editor: Dragan Ilic
ISBN: 978-1-62081-538-0

Chapter 7

Academic and Scientific Poster Presentation - Visualising Knowledge as a Means to Facilitate Knowledge Transfer

Nicholas E. Rowe*
Freelance Academic Writer and Editor - Pello, Finland

Abstract

Poster presentations are a common-place feature of many modern academic and professional settings. Based upon the wide range of professional groups that utilise the medium and the multitude of local, national and international meetings at which they are presented, it may be fair to estimate that millions are undertaken every year. As a stand-alone medium however, they are not best suited to facilitate knowledge transfer. This chapter looks at how we can make the most of the many opportunities for poster presentation and use facilitated dialogue to increase the potential to communicate our findings, opinions and research to others. In particular, it considers those aspects of knowledge transfer commonly found in both the business and conference setting; namely the concepts of knowledge / research dissemination and its subsequent utilization by the receiver. In considering these aspects, this chapter looks to demonstrate that although the academic poster is a favoured medium of visualising knowledge, there are further considerations to be made, if we are to effectively transfer that knowledge to others.

Introduction

If the purpose of this chapter were to discuss the effective knowledge transfer potential of the academic / scientific poster as a stand-alone medium, then it would be very short indeed. The capacity of a 2D visual medium to attract interest or convey a limited message is evident in our everyday lives (e.g. advertisements, branding and signage), but to develop this into a meaningful mechanism of in-depth knowledge transfer, requires additional elements to be

* E-mail address: editorinchief@thewrittenword.eu

considered. No robust empirical studies have been conducted into the actual level of knowledge transfer achieved by the standard poster medium [1,5], which is surprising, given the number of presentations that are given each year. Considering the fields in which they are commonly used (i.e. healthcare, science, medicine, education) and the number of potential conferences at which they are presented, the number of posters compiled must run into millions, yet nobody has measured if they actually work.

Within business, industry and the professional setting, the concepts of knowledge sharing, networking and professional development are well established. Mostly, these are facilitated by means of conferences and symposia at which delegates either present or attend the latest topics within their discipline [1,2,3]. There is a general expectation for professionals to present and publish their work, [4,5] for which these gatherings provide an excellent platform by which this may be achieved. Selecting an appropriate event is important not only in finding a receptive target audience but also realistically, those people "whom you wish to influence" [4]. The motivation to disseminate knowledge (and the egotistic motivation to become the source of that knowledge) remains passive though, unless we seek to influence our prospective audience and in-concept, 'sell' our ideas [5].

These concepts hold parallels with the organizational management aspects of knowledge transfer, around which much of the extant literature emanates and revolves. These exchanges may be likened to 'trade' – a type of '*quid pro quo'* by which all parties seek to gain a mutual benefit. The commodity itself (knowledge), may be contextualised as "… the *acquisition* of data or information. Sometimes it is not new knowledge but *confirmation* of past information" [6]. This later aspect of confirmation implies a need for interaction on a more personal level with the information giver, which is not readily promoted by either didactic lecture or a standalone poster which simply presents data. We are unlikely to simply 'believe' something, just because we hear or see it once and we need a personal understanding and context for it to be meaningful and of use. In order to embed knowledge, it must first be evaluated, tested and contextualised by the receiver, and again this points to the importance of some form of interaction on a personal level.

An original description of a poster as "…a visual combination of bold design, colour and message intended to catch and hold the attention of the passerby long enough to *implant a significant idea in the mind*." [7], may be enough to stimulate some initial interest, but is unlikely to result in the implementation of the displayed knowledge unless pursued further. If we are to enable our findings or research to be effectively utilised, we must ensure that we give the recipient a chance to internalise the information and transfer it to his or her area of interest. This may be best achieved through reciprocal communication and interactive dialogue and poster presentations are an ideal facilitator of this.

Poster Presentation Practices

The dissemination of new research knowledge (or knowledge transfer), is often facilitated by oral, poster and workshop presentations. Where didactic lectures and workshops focus primarily on oral transmission, the academic / scientific poster is essentially seen as a visual medium [1]. Traditional views have maintained that "A poster should speak for itself, without any additional explanation by the presenter" [8], and further, that "… posters show, not tell"

[9]. This has perhaps led to the commonly held misconception, that it is the poster itself that is of central importance in such settings and not the overall presentation and discussion of data. Much of the extant literature and guidance focuses upon the composition and aesthetics of the medium [1,5,10] but there is little on the conversational exchanges themselves, which form an essential element of knowledge transfer in this presentational practice.

Since 2007, reported internet searches for the terms “research poster” or “poster presentation of research” have escalated from around 20,000 hits [10] to millions, indicating the high level of interest in the topic.. Poster presentations are accepted as a genre within academic activity [1,5,10], yet still suffer from a stigma as being a ‘lesser presentation’[10]. In 2004 the US Court of Appeal ruled that a poster presentation depicting a scientific concept was deemed ‘‘to foster general knowledge“ of the subject concerned and so constituted a genuine form of publication [11].

The idea of ‘fostering general knowledge’ however does not push the ultimate aims of knowledge transfer; those of knowledge/research utilization and its subsequent implementation. Knowledge has been described as not merely a collection of data, but “… a person’s ability to *use and apply* information” [10], so this links the commonly applied frameworks of Knowledge Transfer, Evidence-Based Practice and Research Utilization which share such aims.

Most poster literature stems from the backgrounds of healthcare and science [1,5,10], but increasingly, the parallels between these frameworks are being noted [15]. Nursing was an early area in which literature was found, albeit mainly qualitative in nature but medicine and other healthcare professions have also made significant contributions, which are becoming more robust in nature. It is apparent that there is a receptive audience to the medium and it is a popular method by which to disseminate findings, but the actual exchange of information (leading to the creation of knowledge) is little explored.

Knowledge is often personal and affected by individual experience, which makes it difficult to enable others to use directly. To simply present a poster full of data (i.e. explicit knowledge) is therefore not enough – we need to highlight the central concepts of what we have to say and then promote the opportunity for *our* own experience (or tacit knowledge), to be contextualised against that of the receiver.

Poster presentation may not be conducive to 'active learning', although it still meets the expressed professional demand for a 'snap-shot' overview [1]. Unsupported poster presentations may promote some level of active learning, in that the audience must engage with the poster to read, synthesise and analyse the information presented [2,3], but this increases the need for visual themes that attract viewer attention[1] and relies on the commitment of the viewer to ‘stay with’ the poster until they have reached what they perceive to be an adequate level of understanding.

As far as clear-cut ‘facts’ are concerned, the poster can present them clearly and succinctly, yet what of the more qualitative facets – those factors which influence us and what we experience whilst undertaking the work? We cannot transfer the explicitly personal aspects of experiential knowledge to others but we can “transfer the framework or facts upon which that experience is founded”, [10] and this may be best achieved through dialogue. In the academic / scientific setting, it enables the analysis, synthesis and evaluation of information [16], as well as fulfilling those socialisation elements which promote knowledge transfer [12].

Poster presentations may be accompanied by a short presentation (only a few minutes in duration) [10], which serve to alert viewers to what is available to view and to outline salient facts. More commonly however, they are simply amassed in a large area, where people are faced with row upon row of A1 sheets, pinned to boards. The presence of the author during viewing slots, can facilitate discussion between them and the audience yet these timings often compete with breaks from the plenary lectures and sessions and again affects the commitment to learning of both presenter and delegates alike.

The perceived hierarchy of oral presentations over poster presentations has prompted the view that "The academic hierarchy requires that students work their way up to earn the privilege of a captive audience." [10]. Attendees naturally may find the potential wisdom of a pre-eminent speaker more engaging; however, if the subject topic is of little interest then the audience is indeed captive. With poster events the viewer makes a conscious decision to engage with a particular presenter and their work, despite the common lure of food, coffee and the social aspects of the event. The least we can do therefore is to try to ensure that our presentation imparts enough information and context, for the viewer to have gained meaningfully from the exchange.

The poster presentation is more than the physical data on the poster, "it can also be studied as a situated practice" [10]. This is often seen as a challenging aspect of presentation and requires a distinct set of skills and abilities. Explicit knowledge can be transferred by text or verbalization, so the idea of 'data' being 'data' holds true in poster representation – tell it how it is (albeit in an abbreviated form).

Our more tacit knowledge (that which reflects our contexts and experiences), is often not explicitly known and therefore difficult to transfer to users. To attempt a concise description would be immensely challenging (and lead to a text-heavy poster), so ideas and concepts are better introduced or alluded to by a visual stimulus that can prompt the required discussion.

An example may be riding a bicycle – could you simply put the requisite actions on a poster and expect an unknown variety of viewers to be able to then competently peddle off into the sunset? Even if you put the instructions in diagrammatic form; if the aim is to enable viewers to cycle, they are still likely to need some description and perhaps even demonstration, or practical assistance.

Many less experienced presenters view the medium as being more difficult to do well than the traditional written article [10] or standard oral presentation [14], and the issues of communication and knowledge transfer highlighted, may serve to demonstrate why this is so. Contradicting this however, many articles discuss poster presentation as being in the apprentice / student arena and this may emanate from the perception of poster presentations as being a 'lesser' medium of publication, yet there is more to the genre than just a 'pretty picture [1,2,5,8,9,13].

"Learning to communicate research well through posters involves far more than formatting issues and complexity arises from the multiple roles that posters must fulfil" [10]. If we consider the medium to be conducted as an *ad-hoc* oral presentation, advertised and supported by a poster illustrating key points, then we may not only be better prepared for what is to come, but we may also have greater potential to achieve a genuine transfer of knowledge.

Perhaps these activities would be better described in the future as 'Poster Supported Presentations', with a clear prescriptive requirement published by event organisers of what is expected from presenters.

The Viewing Process – Visual Aspects of Poster Presentation

Attracting a viewer's attention is the first visual objective of the poster medium. A viewer will see the poster from a distance, long before they are able to read its title or text. Unless you have an audience, you have no one to talk to. An event participant in a UK study stated: "The poster medium is an excellent discipline for crystallizing your views on a topic. However unless you get a chance to discuss the poster with other delegates it can feel like you are having a discourse with yourself" [1]. In this instance, the principles of sales and advertising apply - if there is nobody in your store, there is nobody to buy your product, so attract them into the 'zone'.

Attracting Attention - from Non-Participant to Bystander

A large, centrally placed image is more likely to attract the eye, than a series of closely written text boxes [5]. We are attracted more to difference than similarity, so the more innovative or creative posters tend to stand out (in Figure 1, did you look at the two blank triangles or focus on the shaded one?). The cry 'gimmick' rings out, yet it is a key fact that successful posters will have high impact visual components. If we consider roadside advertising, which are we best able to recall; the emotive or shocking images of high-end advertising campaigns or the text informing us of a super, low-cost garage sale next Saturday? The fact that we are 'advertising' our work, should not stir out-dated sentiments on the status of 'trade', so these principles should be embraced (after all, most of the initial concepts of knowledge transfer came from the business setting).

Everyday technology allows us to create highly visual posters [1,5,10], so there is little excuse for creating something that looks more like the closely-packed columns of a news paper. The idea of billboard advertising is to perhaps sell a product, the idea of the garage sale sign is to get you to come and possibly buy something. The idea of advertising in an academic / scientific poster is to get you to engage in discourse around a subject and effect knowledge sharing and transfer. Imagery has been seen to hold an 'interactional metafunction' [28], specifically in creating a warmer atmosphere in which dialogue can take place. This first stage observation allows the viewer to create his / her own mental concept of what may lie ahead and align themselves with the envisaged topic. Think of road signs warning of men at work or a low bridge ahead – we see the image and conceptualize the potential danger, before we are close enough to read the description that accompanies the sign.

Our visual perception allows rapid judgements to be made that can then be confirmed and verified by words (oral or written). Images appeal to our emotions and help people to in effect, 'see' what we mean. As well as catching attention, they may inspire or stimulate thought in viewers that can then be capitalized upon to initiate dialogue. From a learning perspective, they improve recall and facilitate learning [29] as the viewer assimilates the image to their own perspective. When images are used interactively, they can help to support reasoning and communication, which again promotes their usage in the knowledge transfer setting. In Figure 2 are two examples of posters, which view differently from afar. At a distance of 20 meters (simulated), both are generally unreadable, yet the colour of the image on the top and the size/emotiveness of the image on the bottom, stand out.

When viewed closely, it is the right hand image that is likely to be most memorable, because of its size, focal position and lack of explicit linkage or detail. As the image is not predefined, we are free to link it with our own meanings and attributions, which also personalises it to us and makes it more meaningful. This mental linkage acts as a tool to our construct of knowledge and gives us a visual 'hook', on which to hang different aspects of the subject information. In the same way that the 'hook' drew us towards the poster initially, it can also help us retrieve information in the future, which aids knowledge recall and increases the potential for its future use.

Written words also stimulate visual mental responses and help to create a framework of ideas, upon which we can crystallize knowledge. Examples from the passage on road signs (above) may be *'first stage'* which sub-consciously prompts the idea that there is a second stage to be reached and draws you mentally forward. '*create ... [a] mental concept*' grants you freedom to think for yourself and adapt what you see, whilst *'what may lie ahead'* can entice you to picture or imagine the immediate future. Written words are however not reciprocal and lack the para-verbal affirmations that help to support learning through oral dialogue, so a combination of spoken and written words and imagery is required. Although used in the context of poster compilation, the phrase which conjures "images of attaching words to ideas as they start to gel, building an infrastructure, and hanging concepts on a framework" [10], gives not only a mental image of a poster taking shape, but also an anticipation of the constructive dialogue that may stem from interacting with a poster presentation. In this, the use of selected wording or imagery can help attract viewers and initiate dialogue, which again, is the first objective of poster presentation.

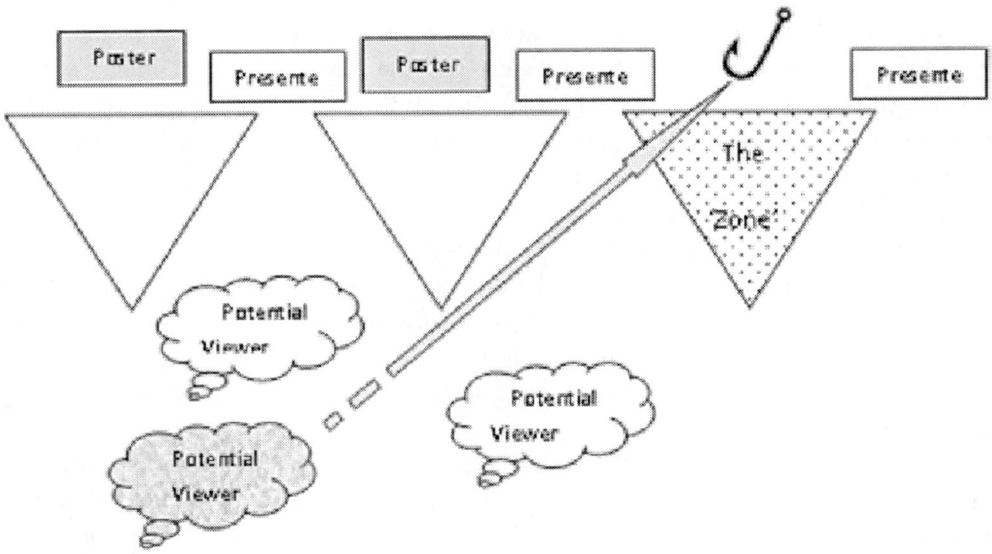

Figure 1. Visual attraction at poster viewing sessions the key to initiating dialogue.

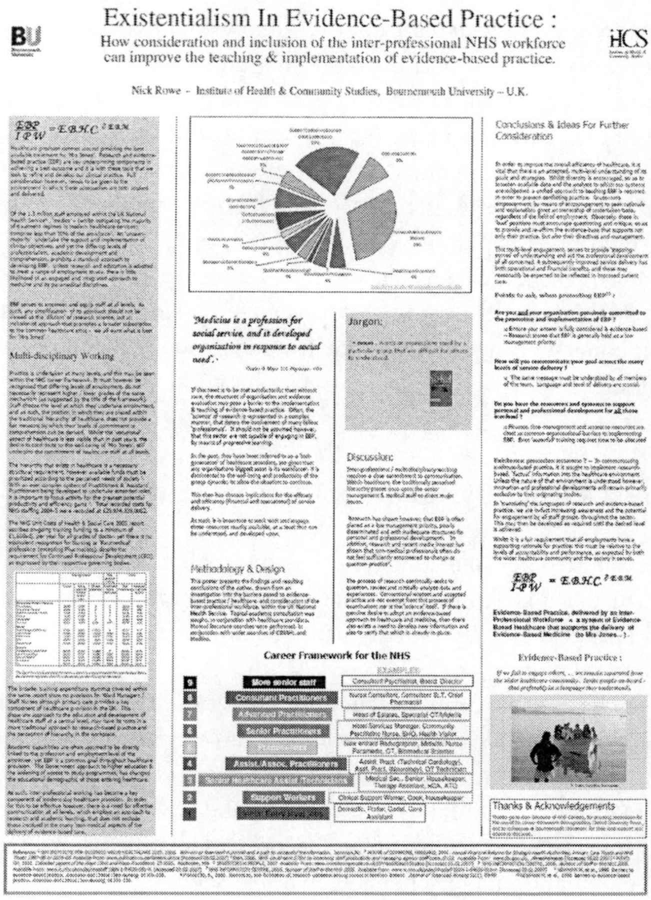

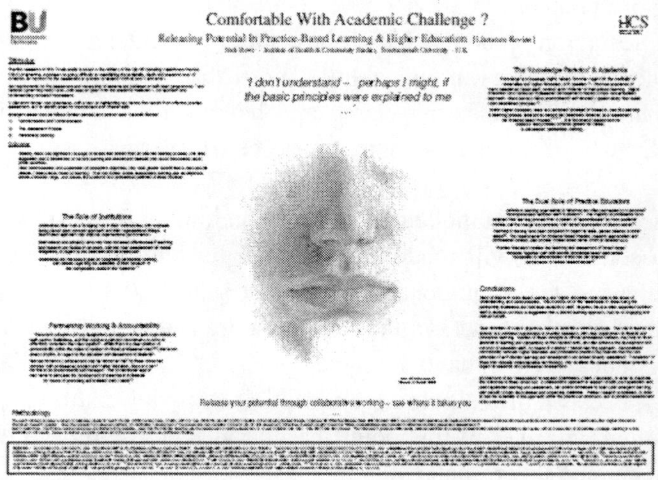

(Top image [33]) Rowe, N., 2007. Existentialism in Evidence-Based Practice: How consideration and inclusion of the inter-professional workforce can improve the teaching and implementation of evidence-based practice.

(Bottom image [34]) Rowe, N., 2007. Comfortable With Academic Challenge? Releasing Potential in Practice-Based Learning and Higher Education [Literature Review].

Figure 2. A1 Poster imagery, when viewed from a distance of 20 meters (simulated).

As a visual conception, objects can help to attract attention [29] and enhance learning. They appeal to the haptic domain and also aid communication. Envisage the first time you hold a 35 million year old dinosaur fossil (as opposed to just see it in a case) or lay your hand on a beating human heart during surgery (as opposed to simply seeing the image in a book); the added dimension of tactile memory or perception, greatly enhances both the learning experience and the deeper conceptualization of the learning moment. Of course, the level of appropriateness of the object should be considered (i.e. giant blow up rabbit or touch-screen technology?), but the presence of physical things can serve to both attract the attention of potential viewers and initiate discussion. However we chose to do so, our aim is to turn a passer-by, into someone who approaches the fringe of our presentational 'zone', with the possible intent of interacting.

Taking an Interest - from Bystander to Passive Participant

As the viewer approaches the zone, he becomes able to read the title of the work. Naturally, the size of the text is larger so that it can be read from outside the zone, from a distance of around 5 meters and again, may use a combination of font and colour differences to continue to attract attention.

The wording needless to say, must accurately reflect the key content and direction of the topic covered, but again, there is scope for creative neuro-linguistic phrasing that continues to attract the attention of the viewer.

If again, this smacks of 'gimmick', then consider the wordy, colon-riddled titles of many journal articles – you have to be chosen as the presenter with whom the viewer wants to interact and emotive text and imagery helps viewers to see your point in a manner which best suits their learning preference.

If a high-end restaurant menu listed dishes simply 'meat and potatoes' or 'fish and cheese', you would rightly be wanting a little more than that to arrive at your table. If however we are partial to for example, lamb and have a good understanding of what the described meal might be like, then we may chose that dish as it is explicit and details its components.

There is no need to feel compelled to drop in random snippets of French or exclusive jargon that only a select few will readily understand, but the title or description has to be appealing to its intended target audience. That being said however, a highly visual person may look across at what other diners in the restaurant are eating and say, 'I don't know what that is, but it looks good, so I will have the same'.

Images though, because of their emotive potential, help viewers to hang their own words or concepts upon them and it is at this point that the viewer is likely to enter the zone and engage with the poster and its presenter.

In the main, viewers will enter the zone and focus firstly on the poster itself. They are at a distance where all of the text should be readable and a quick overview will give them the background knowledge they need, before they 'risk' inter-personal dialogue, more often than not, with someone they do not know.

The formatting and layout of academic / scientific posters is discussed widely in literature and forms the bulk of published discussion [1,5]. Visually, the compilation should remain uncluttered. 'Busy' posters are off-putting to viewers, together with those that are harsh on the eye in regard to colour, font variation and layout.

Only the key points of the work should be highlighted and there should be a logical transition between sections, sign posted if necessary [18,19]. Each section should be clearly titled and again, be designed to promote clarity of understanding. It is important to remember that whilst explicit information (data) transfers well by the spoken or written word, the tacit knowledge we hold often requires interactive communication.

As such, issues should be briefly (but clearly) referred to on the poster with visual prompts and representations where appropriate. The intent is to provide a comprehensive *overview* of the topic and not to foster an in-depth knowledge of the issues involved, so again, clarity is the key.

From the viewers standpoint, there is a limited element of active learning involved as they analyze, synthesize and evaluate information [1] but it is not reciprocal interaction, when compared to standard models [20,21].

The essence of tacit issues and deeper levels of information should be transferred through discourse between the presenter and what have now become the participants. To aid this, further use of additional material, hyperlinked electronic data and multi-media sources can be used, either built into a digitally presented 'Media Poster' style presentation or simply as adjunct materials and resources [32].

It is not uncommon though to have a person approach your presentation and say 'That's a really nice looking poster ... so what's it all about then?' (cue strong visual learning preference). Whatever people's motivation for approaching your work, they are now engaged with you on a learning level, so you need to interact positively with them.

Interaction and Achieving Knowledge Transfer

Reciprocal Communication – The Key to Active Participation

The tri-partite structure of poster presentation components (poster, presenter and viewer – Figure 3) is mirrored in work which analysed the conversational participation structure at poster presentation events [17]. It identified a 'conversational space' (similar to the triangular zone depicted in Figure 1), in which interactions took place. Specifically, they noted that people participated in or entered the area in front of the poster, either to listen to the presenter or view the poster more closely. They could also further participate in the presentation by entering into the conversation itself. The study identifies a progression of audience members from non-participant to bystander; from bystander to side participant (where their presence is noted by others); from side participant to addressee (where they are directly addressed by the speaker) and finally, from addressee to speaker, in which role they address other participants.

They note that these role progressions require sanctioning by other participants in the presentation and so the presenter also takes on a facilitative role [17]. Without this function being met, the poster would remain a restricted medium, in terms of knowledge transfer potential. Picking up on cues from the participant, "the presenter has to be adept at moving between levels of detail and stages of the research as portrayed in the poster, which requires a high degree of flexibility, familiarity with the study, and knowledge of the research" [10].

The transfer of narrative during the conversations utilizes guided experience to inform and re-affirm the key points of the work to the participant. As previously mentioned, tacit aspects of organizational and experiential knowledge can be difficult to represent succinctly. It is recognised however, that organisations can affect knowledge transfer by embedding knowledge in interactions that involve people [22] and reciprocal dialogue is the most effective method of transferring tacit knowledge.

Verbal exchanges focus on the use of language. This has a special role in effecting knowledge transfer, by allowing information to be exchanged and concurrently building on the social exchange which in turn strengthens bonds between those involved [23]. Reciprocal communication brings about shared understandings and helps to contextualise the work against the situation or thinking of the participant. Particularly, the process of language alignment [20] plays a major role in achieving this.

The process of questioning and response allows details of the work presented to be contextualised and tested by the participant. If there is no reciprocal dialogue, then the participant remains effectively a viewer, as confirmation cannot be actively sought and issues are merely taken at face value. Figure 4 illustrates the process of enquiry, from its initial instigation and exchanges, until a confirmed understanding has been reached. As can be seen, the poster acts as a facilitative tool which can present specific data items, or as a focus point upon which to crystallize lines of enquiry. If there are integral points which are key to the enquiry, then these may be referred to on the poster however most of the understanding and knowledge transfer is achieved by interactive conversational dialogue.

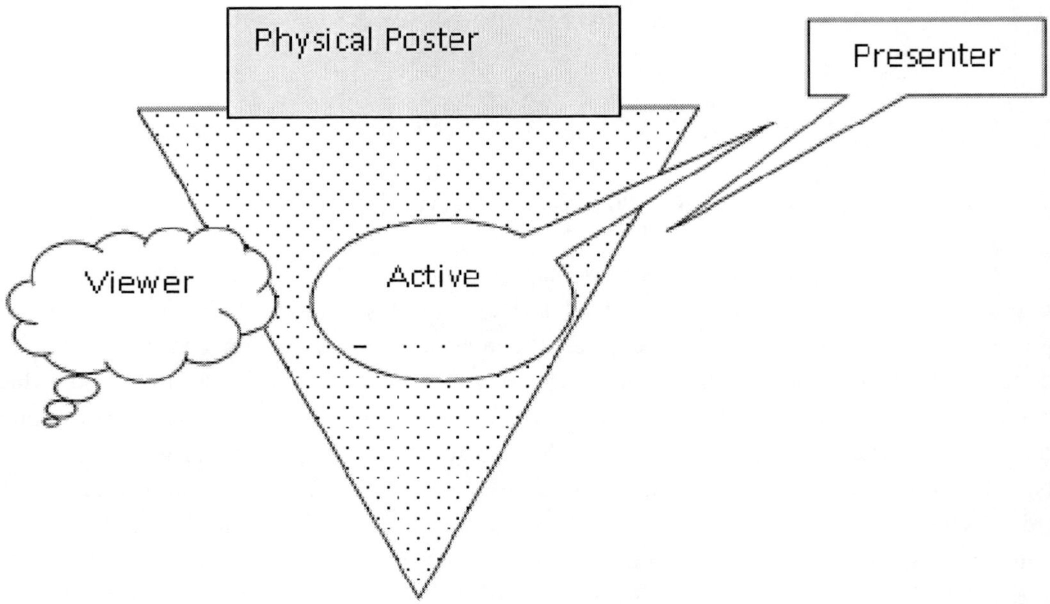

Figure 3. The situational components of interactive poster presentation.

In using spoken language to convey information, we align both the presenter and participant against the context of the work portrayed. Stage 1 of Figure 4 represents the initial contact and exchange between the participant and the presenter.

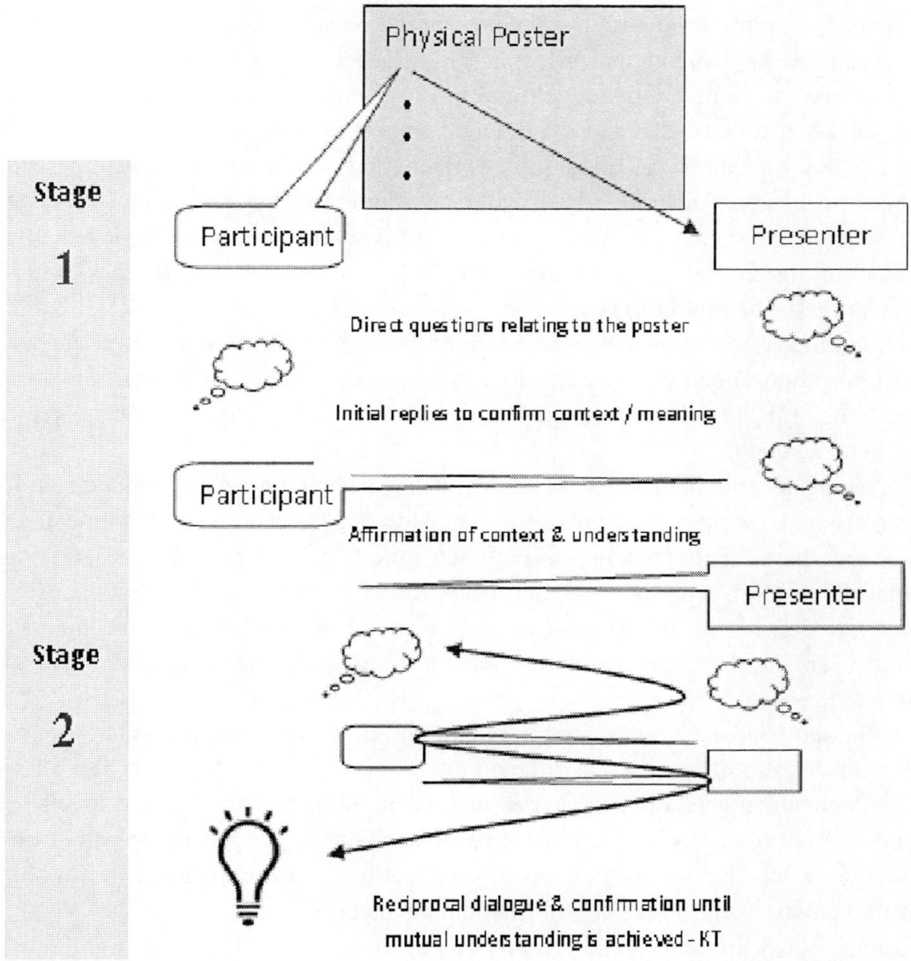

Figure 4. Reciprocal dialogue to achieve understanding and knowledge transfer in the poster presentation setting: a three stage model.

The participant asks formal questions, seeking to guage the content of the poster and their potential ability to interact with the presenter. Questions are mainly closed in format, as we look to establish a conceptual framework on which to build knowledge on the subject. It is during these early stages that most references to the specific aspects of the poster will be made.

"… learning by talking also involves language coordination" [20] and we learn to appreciate the terms which people use to express their thoughts and experiences. In Stage 2 of the model, the participants knowledge framework construction becomes more focused. At this stage, not only are we likely to discuss a specific domain but we also explain to the other party, what we mean by it [20] and importantly, what it means to us.

In doing so, we learn about explicit facts, together with the experiential or tacit background against which they are set. This helps to convey our experiences to others in a more complete way and the dialogue evolves into a more open exchange, as we come to appreciate the knowledge and experience the other party has to offer, as being of potential benefit to ourselves.

The misconception or non-understanding of tacit elements of a work, poses a key barrier to the subsequent implementation of transferred knowledge. This is often down to the initial construct of the recipient's knowledge framework, where they often understand the 'facts' of an issue, but are unable to identify with them on a personal level.

An example of this is the 'hard sell' we sometimes meet in stores: we appreciate how good the product or service is, but need our own time and space to match its features and price to our circumstances, or perhaps make a comparison to other products. If we are interrupted in forming this 'knowledge-base', then we may not have the confidence or inclination to take the sale further.

Both participant (customer) and presenter (salesman) have their own angles on the information (product) being presented, so a mutual understanding has to be developed. This helps to transform the information into embedded knowledge upon which judgements and decisions can be made.

In learning to communicate with each other, we develop a shared understanding. We share words and become 'in-step' with the ways we relate and communicate and this enhances our shared understanding on both semantic and conceptual levels [20]. Stage 3 of the model (Figure IV), represents a reciprocal phase of dialogue in which both participant and presenter are aligned. By this stage, the main areas of the presentation are understood and both parties are now seeking to embed the knowledge and open up alternative areas for consideration.

The dialogue becomes more open in nature and participant and presenter both recognise what the other has to offer, placing value on their tacit experience. There is also an increased level of tolerance between differing styles of speech and para-verbal usage, together with an acceptance of impressionistic issues, such as perhaps dress, personality or perceived aspects of professionalism. This acceptance is self-propagating, and in-turn leads to a more relaxed and trusting environment, in which information can be exchanged.

Neuro-linguistically we can add to this by mirroring the immediate learning preferences, demonstrated by the participant. Conformational phrases like 'I see what you mean', 'I feel that …', 'I hear what you are saying' etc, can indicate how an individual may benefit from illustrative examples, elaboration of the qualitative concepts or perhaps just further explanation. This promotes effective knowledge transfer and leads from a short, direct line of questioning, to a more open and shared discussion.

Additionally, it aids the participant's memory retention and thus increases their potential to utilize the knowledge in the future. The observation of body language also helps to direct dialogue, although there is a common misconception that every movement or pose is a firm representation of how the person is feeling or receiving the situation. We do however, tend to measure this sub-consciously and it helps to observe signs of understanding, relaxation and commitment during presentations.

This can be helpful in the simplest of circumstances; for example, if the participant is genuinely interested in the subject, but is also competing with the urge for caffeine, there is no reason why you can't continue the conversation over coffee – a little empathy goes a long way. Interactions at this level promote a social cohesion and willingness of individuals to collaborate in the sharing and development of knowledge [23]. In the conference setting, this may apply to a wide range of individuals with a variety of backgrounds, and the potential uses for the transferred knowledge are many. Each dialogue participant can take the core principles of the work discussed and examine its relation to his / her specialist field.

The result is an expanded network that draws from a common theme, yet is able to diversify to meet the needs of individual members.

Often, this progresses into a shared understanding of the wider application of the work discussed and can lead to future collaboration. This relationship between individuals is identified as a key component of effective knowledge transfer [10,30,31] and an expressed aim of conference attendance [5] .

ISSUES ENCOUNTERED IN POSTER PRESENTATION AND DIALOGUE

Knowledge is often confused with 'training' and the instilling of un-tested facts. The presentation of data and experiences using the poster medium, promotes the opportunity to explore these 'facts', until a shared understanding is reached. Current perceptions of quality and esteem however, continue to denigrate the genre [1,2,5,10]. From their earliest stages, posters have been viewed by some quarters as being non-specific and as such 'unsophisticated' [24]. Perhaps this 'vagueness' is because issues are not actively transmitted to any depth as people often expect the medium to act in an almost stand alone capacity [1,5,10]. If we re-visit the bicycle analogy mentioned earlier, then it is hardly surprising that those who expect to ride a bike solely on the instructions portrayed on a poster, suffer a few cuts and bruises as a result.

The poster itself is required to have key informational components that illustrate the work presented. As such, it can give an overall snapshot and act as a facilitative prop, around which to focus discussion. The emphasis of these presentations however, is to communicate information and experience, so that they become usable knowledge for others. All the important facets of your work cannot be feasibly included on the poster itself, so it is crucial to decide what to include and what to omit [25]. In this, the poster 'machines' the research material [10] to give a concise overview, around which discussions can take place. This is however an acquired skill and such an overly succinct writing style does not always come readily to authors.

Highlighted points form the framework upon which the argument or issue is built, with images or visual aids helping to provide further implicit infrastructure. The material that perhaps more 'existentialist' critics may simply view as being absent, should be readily provided by the presenter. Again, they can refer to the indicative imagery of the poster, to convey some of the more tacit experiences and issues.

This requires presenters to move knowledgeably in and out of elements of the poster, in a way that is controlled by the needs and understanding of the participant, and not a pre-planned format that can be rehearsed and polished by the presenter [10,14]. As such, an in-depth familiarity with the content and mechanisms of the work is essential [5].

Historically, authors are often not available to their prospective audience at convenient times [10,26] and may be ill-prepared for in-depth questioning on their subject. A balance has to be struck between the presenter's desire to present material to as many others as possible, and their own needs in attending such dissemination events. It must though be said, that in undertaking such a presentation, the posters author has an obligation to meet the needs of others as far as is reasonably possible. To this end, some organizers are starting to include platform presentations to introduce poster topics and laid down requirements regarding the availability of presenters during poster viewing sessions [10].

As a poster presenter, you are often exposed to random and varying lines of enquiry, as participants seek to align their understanding of your work, with their own contextual background. Learning simply by observing a presentation or viewing a poster has limitations, so the participant is likely to demand more than is immediately on display.

To this end, there is a requirement not only for a thorough knowledge of the subject, but also for diverse skills such as empathy, facilitation and communication. Add to that the artistic and compositional skills involved in the creation of the poster itself and it becomes apparent that the poster genre is in-fact, not for the feint-hearted. Visual literacy is important in attracting the viewer and also helps to illustrate tacit elements of the work, but for presentations to be successful and robust, the role of the presenter is key.

Interaction during poster presentations is vital to achieving knowledge transfer, not only through the clarification of information, but also in the creation of knowledge networks. Attendees at conferences are often individuals from a range of backgrounds that work within what they view as the cultural norms of their institutions and their experience. In participating in the socialization and acculturation that such gatherings engender, attendees begin to see alternative ways of operating within their own fields, as well as sharing new knowledge with others. It is a recognized business fact that the stronger a company's links and networks are, the more profitable it is likely to be. Transposed to the academic / scientific arena, this suggests that both the individual and their institution stand to benefit from interaction, however this needs to exceed the niceties of coffee and a brief chat, and take the form of genuine reciprocal dialogue, as depicted in Figure 3, centered upon a topic of mutual interest. Poster presentations are often taken as 'fillers' for peoples time, so the willingness of attendees to engage in reciprocal dialogue is sometimes limited and this results in ineffective knowledge transfer.

The embedded knowledge that many bring to the initial phases of a discussion, can reflect many of the known constrains of the workplace, including systematic thinking and routines, the relationships between professional roles, and formal procedures [10]. People may have pre-conceived ideas about what the poster should contain or perhaps how the information is presented. The political issues surrounding 'knowledge' may manifest themselves as differences in opinion and practice, levels of perceived expertise or maybe the transferability of context and application, and these can all have an adverse impact on the initial exchanges and impressions that are created during the initial phases of the presentation. Coming from a range of backgrounds and working cultures, all too often, we impose the 'facts' of our own practice and experience, as the normal or expected practice of the wider community. This introduces a potentially 'hostile' or alien element to presenting [27] and changes the environment from something more removed (such as a journal article or podium lecture where responses are less instantaneous), to a more intimate and personal setting. Pursuing a reciprocal dialogue approach however, helps both parties in sharing the socialisation process that involved in achieving mutual understanding and effective knowledge transfer.

The issue of poster (*sic.* publication) replication is also an issue raised in literature [1,10]. Posters are not readily distributed in hard format due to their size and cost in production. The abstracts of presentations are readily available at most events, yet the format is often even more constrained than the poster itself, in terms of what it can meaningfully convey. To have only 250 or 300 words is not uncommon whereas an uncluttered and succinct poster can easily have upwards of 1000 [5], so there is little representation of the actual depth of the presentation or work itself. Poster presentations are considered a valid form of publication [1,5] but as they are not 'published' in the same sense as a journal article, there are concerns that authors receive multiple credit (as citations on their CV), for trundling the same poster around different event venues [10]. Whether the poster presentation is CV or KT motivated, it is often viewed as less robustly considered (if at all) by peer review and as such seen as an 'easy' way to score a 'publication'. This judgement is unfortunately often applied to many who choose to undertake the genre.

THE WAY FORWARD

As things currently stand, there is too little emphasis on the presentational aspects and skills of effective poster presentations and their potential for active knowledge transfer. Re-branding the medium as 'Poster Supported Presentations', would bring the communicative aspects of presentation to the fore and potentially effect a greater degree of knowledge transfer than has previously been recognised. The medium is currently well equipped to achieve this:

- the knowledge holders are present
- they are motivated to share with an audience that favours the medium
- the use of Posters as a facilatory tool is a good transfer mechanism

Organizers of events should provide clear guidelines as to what they expect from presenters and how they in-turn will manage the event. They should establish whether posters have been presented at other events in the past and at what level, and if so, request a justification from the author as to why their work should be considered for acceptance at a second event.

The knowledge transfer plan of poster presentations is all too often a random event with competing interests, e.g. a coffee break or 'free time' during which participants (including presenters) either wish to eat, socialize or simply need a break from proceedings. Given the level of work that is required to affect a good poster presentation, the skills involved and the sheer number of posters which are delivered each year, then more consideration and uniformity is needed in how such events are managed. The current use of short introductory oral presentations helps to highlight the topics that people can engage with and removes some of the random browsing that often occurs, but there is still the question of interaction, in what is essentially a voluntary or open attendance presentation.

If funded by an institution or external body, presenters (of all types of format), should compile a reflective account of their experience, which details their interactions, thoughts and future considerations. This can then be made available internally within their organizations, so that others may benefit and learn from what they have experienced. The socialization process is also a key part of conference attendance and integral to network building, so institutions should consider this aspect of 'return' and again expect some form of feedback which considers this element. It may also include coverage of how the event and presentations attended, may tie in to future work and development. On a personal level, this practice helps to analyze and contextualize our experiences, so the benefits to both institution and individual are mutual. Again another business parallel, but many successful businessmen keep a diary or reflective journal which helps them capitalize on events – there is no reason why this practice cannot transfer to other settings where individuals need to reflect on information, in order to give a greater potential for its integration in future work.

In providing a link to presentations and their impact upon future work, it may be easier to address two clearly missing elements of knowledge transfer within the poster genre, and they are knowledge utilization and implementation. Some minor studies have touched upon the perception and experiences of those presenting posters at events [1,10] and many of the respondents in the studies felt that (their) posters were of a sufficient robustness to stand alone. The posters efficacy as a medium of knowledge transfer however remains only conjecture as no specific measurement of transfer or application has been undertaken. Those who 'judge' poster presentations are often happy with a representation of facts, which are quick to read, clearly presented and need little if no elaboration – they do not however consider the more tacit elements of many forms of knowledge that are involved in many works, especially those around many of the disciplines which utilize the medium (e.g. health and social care or medicine) and so may be confusing knowledge with 'data' or information. To re-cap, knowledge is a personal concept that revolves around an individual's ability to *use and apply* information.

That said; the measurement of *knowledge transfer* (which after all, is a prime objective of knowledge communication and sharing) has to consider not only if the information has been received clearly (as established in reciprocal dialogue) but also if it has been effectively utilized.

If we have lots of 'facts' floating around in our heads, we could certainly be of use to the local quiz team and have a certain 'smugness' regarding our own capacity to remember things. To be of use to a broader element of society however, then we need to bring these facts out and utilize them in a more meaningful and focused way. Posters are an established and popular medium by which to present knowledge but further work needs to be undertaken to develop their presentational delivery. The highlighted principles of exploratory dialogue within knowledge transfer and the reported 'loneliness' of poster presenters, would suggest that participant interaction is not being utilized effectively and as such, limits the potential for effective knowledge transfer and utilization. It is only through this development that we can further refine the medium to make it more than just a pretty picture.

REFERENCES

[1] N. Rowe and D. Ilic. *BMC Medical Education*, 9 (71); 1472-6920. (2009).

[2] J. Berg. *J. of the American Academy of Nurse Practitioners*, 17; 245-8. (2005).

[3] S. Duchin and G. Sherwood. *J. of Continuing Education in Nursing*; 21; 205-8. (1990).

[4] M. Cleary and G. Walter. *International J. of Mental Health Nursing,* 13; 204-207. (2004).

[5] N. Rowe and D. Ilic. *J. of Paediatric Respiratory Reviews*, 12; 208-213. (2011).

[6] A. Mumford. *The Learning Organization*, 1 (1); 4-10. (1994).

[7] W. Wittich and C. Schuller. *Instructional technology: Its nature and use*. Harper and Row, New York. (1973).
[8] C. Russell, D. Gregory, and M. Gates. *Qualitative Health Research,* 6 (4); 542-52. (1996).
[9] V. Miracle and K. Cassidy King. *Applied Nursing Research,* 7 (3); 147-157. (1994).
[10] A. MacIntosh-Murray. *Science Communication*, 28 (3); 347-376. (2007).
[11] B. Adams and J. Patrea Pabst. *Tissue Engineering*, 10; 1841–2. (2004).
[12] G. Guzman. *J. of Workplace Learning*, 20 (3); 195-212. (2008).
[13] S. Walker. *J. of Family Therapy*, 27; 285-288. (2005).
[14] P. Martin. *Applied Nursing Research* 7 (4); 208-10. (1994).
[15] D. Orendorff, A. Ramirez and E. Coakes. *Studies in Health Technology Information*, 137; 116-29. (2008).
[16] K. Hyland. *J. of Pragmatics,* 30 (4); 437-55. (1998).
[17] M. Bono, N. Suzuki and Y. Katagiri. *Human-Computer Interaction - Interact*, 03; 713-716. (2003).
[18] H. Taggert and C. Arslanian. *Orthopedic Nursing*, 19; 47-52. (2000).
[19] A. Butz, L. Kohr and D. Jones. *J. of Pediatric Health Car*, 46; 45-48. (2004).
[20] M. Pickering and S. Garrod. *Behavioral and Brain Sciences*, 27; 212-225. (2004).
[21] J. DeVito. *The Interpersonal Communication Book*. 9th ed. Longman, New York. (2001).
[22] L. Argote and P. Ingram. *Organizational Behaviour and Human Decision Processes*, 82, (1); 150-169. (2000).
[23] R. Reagans and B. McIlvey. *Administrative Science Quarterly*, 48 (2); 240-267. (2003).
[24] B. Dubois. *International Journal of the Sociology of Language* 56; 67-84. (1985).
[25] C. Schryer in; *Genre and the new rhetoric*, A. Freedman and P. Medway eds, 105-124. Taylor and Francis, London. (1994).
[26] J. Brooks-Brunn. *Applied Nursing Research,* 9 (2); 97-9. (1996).
[27] G. Guzman. *Journal of Workplace Learning*, 20 (3); 195-212. (2008).
[28] E. Rowley-Jolivet. *English for Specific Purposes,* 21; 19-40. (2002).
[29] Knowledge Visualization. org. New visual approaches in Business. http://www.knowledge-visualization.org (2008).
[30] D. Remenyi, B. Williams, A. Money and E. Swartz. Doing Research in Business and Management, an Introduction to Process and Methods. Sage, London. (1998).
[31] F. Blackler. *Organization Studies,* 16; 1021. (1995).
[32] N. Rowe and D. Ilic. Medical Education, 43; 471-499. (2009).
[33] Rowe, N. *4th International Conference of Evidence-Based Health Care Teachers and Developers*, Taormina, Italy. (2007).
[34] Rowe, N. *Association for Peri-Operative Practice National Congress,* Harrogate, UK. (2007).

In: Knowledge Transfer: Practices, Types and Challenges
Editor: Dragan Ilic
ISBN: 978-1-62081-538-0

Chapter 8

EVIDENCE BASED GUIDELINE (EBG) DEVELOPMENT: A PRACTICAL GUIDE

Marie L. Misso[1,2,*] and Helena J. Teede[1,3]
[1]School of Public Health and Preventative Medicine, Monash University, Melbourne, Australia
[2]Jean Hailes for Women's Health, Melbourne, Australia
[3]Department of Diabetes, Southern Health, Melbourne, Australia

ABSTRACT

This chapter is a practical guide to developing an evidence based guideline (EBG). It begins with a discussion about EBGs, their place within health information overall, why they are important and why it is important that they are developed in a rigorous and systematic way.

While EBG development guidance is available, there is inconsistency in the amount of detail across this guidance and it has been suggested that practical information to complement existing resources may be helpful.

Therefore, logistics of EBG development and practical step by step information about their development is discussed using an example of a nationally approved EBG in the area of polycystic ovary syndrome (PCOS).

We also provide directions to other helpful resources, tools and templates for each step. Practical concepts covered include establishing a multidisciplinary evidence based guideline development group (EBGDG); clinical question development and prioritisation; evidence review and synthesis; drafting of recommendations; obtaining consensus among the EBGDG; and preparing and finalising the EBG for dissemination.

The authors have no conflicts of interest to declare.

* Corresponding author: E-mail:marie.misso@monash.edu

ACKNOWLEDGMENT

The authors would like to acknowledge Dr. Tari Turner for valuable comments on an earlier version of this chapter.

INTRODUCTION

Health information in the form of guidance about clinical practice can be presented in different formats such as evidence based guidelines (EBGs), non-evidence based clinical practice guidelines, consensus statements, organisation or service provider position statements, systematic reviews, care pathways or algorithms; and by different groups of individuals such as local, national, international groups, public or private sector or combinations, professional societies, public agencies, health care institutions, and researchers. Differences in guidance are largely based on the process used and/or reported to develop them. EBGs follow a specific systematic process to minimise bias that is defined a priori and reported accordingly to be reproducible with conclusions linked to the evidence, whereas non-EBGs may lack rigor, methodology may not be transparent and developers may make recommendations based on a selection of evidence – perhaps based on their own agenda. The rigorous systematic process used in developing EBGs is what makes EBGs trustworthy, reliable and useable and is the subject of this chapter.

The Importance of Methodologically Rigorous EBGs

Traditionally, clinical practice guidelines were not developed using evidence based principles such as strategically searching for, selecting and appraising evidence. Increased adoption of evidence base medicine, encouraged by organisations such as The Cochrane Collaboration, led to the merging of such principles with clinical practice guidelines, the result being EBGs which are now the gold standard for health information. EBGs outline expectations for practice and pathways of care and outline the likely outcomes of care [1].

EBGs also identify gaps in available evidence. The purpose ofEBGs is to integrate the best available evidence with clinical expertise and consumer preferences, to provide health professionals, consumers and policy makers with guidance on a particular topic. They are intended, not to replace, but to aid clinical judgment and patient preference.

Recommendations may relate to a specific population but may not apply to individual patients [2], therefore the ultimate decision about clinical management of an individual patient will always depend on the clinical circumstances, preferences of the patient, and on the clinical judgment of the health care team (Figure 1).

EBGs provide recommendations to guide clinical practice and have the potential to improve patient outcomes, promote standardised care, develop standards to assess the clinical practice of healthcare professionals, support education and training of healthcare professionals, assess healthcare costs and promote research and translation into practice and policy [2, 4, 5].

When a methodologically rigorous development process has been followed, EBGs provide a reliable source of synthesised and appraised information in the one place, providing certainty in clinical practice leads to minimisation of potential harms. Documenting the process transparently is of utmost importance as it allows the reader to have confidence in the recommendations. There has been substantial investment in the development and dissemination of guidelines to inform clinical practice.

Turner and colleagues reported that when the medical subject heading 'practice guideline' was introduced in MEDLINE in 1993, there were 444 articles, by 2006 this number was increased by eleven-fold to 4,975 articles [4].

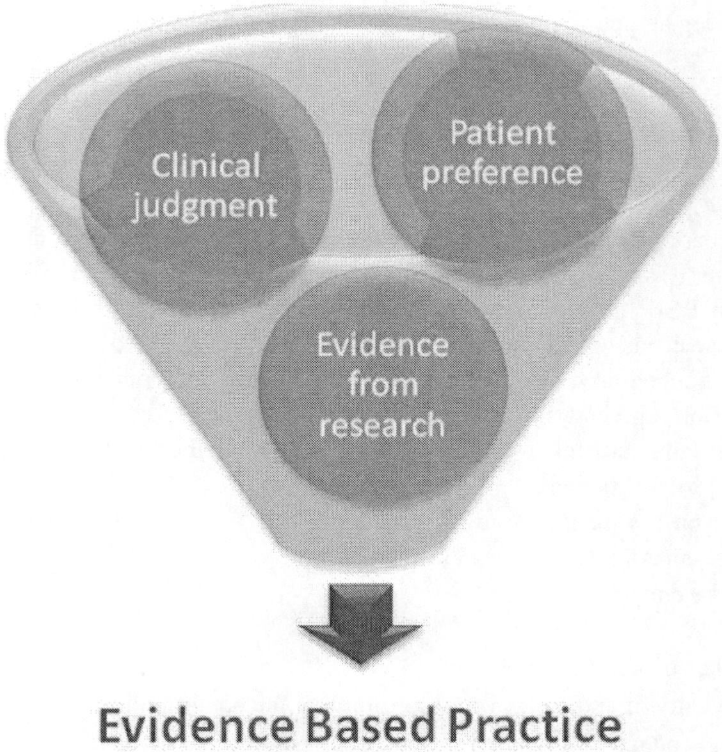

Figure 1.Evidence base practice, reproduced with permission from Teede et al. 2011 [3].

As guideline development methodology has evolved, national and international organisations have increasingly developed their own new guidelines, which has led to multiple guidelines addressing the same topic [6]. The quality and consistency of these guidelines and the evidence used to inform their recommendations vary greatly and is often poor [6-14].

This is of concern for multiple reasons: where guidelines are consistent, the duplication of effort has the potential to be a waste of time and intensive resources; where they are inconsistent, recommendations may be conflicting and facilitate uncertainty in clinical practice [15] or inappropriate care. An exemplar is the uncertainty generated by multiple consensus based guidelines about assessment of the features of PCOS. As a result 70% of women with PCOS remain undiagnosed with resultant lost opportunities for prevention(16).

The implications of flawed clinical guidance is discussed in further detail by Woolf and colleagues [2].

To avoid such implications, guideline development handbooks are available (11, 17-21) and provide relatively consistent advice about the main steps of EBG development [4], however they vary in terms of the type and quantity of detail provided. Many studies have demonstrated a mismatch between recommended methods for development of EBGs and actual methods reported [6, 15, 22-31]. Perhaps more practical detail about the steps listed in these handbooks may be required [4]. Here we provide practical information on the steps of EBG development using an example from the nationally approved *Evidence-based guideline for the assessment and management of polycystic ovary syndrome* (http://www.managingpcos.org.au/pcos-evidence-based-guidelines) at each step[5].

Things to Consider Before Starting the Process of Developing an EBG

Establish Need

Before embarking on the process of developing an EBG, the topic needs to be explored in terms of whether it is a priority for clinical practice, consumers and policy. In establishing the imperative for EBG development, given the substantial investment in time, effort and funding, the case needs to be carefully considered.

If it is not a recognised priority, most guideline endorsing bodies will require significant justification before agreeing to consider a new EBG. Issues to consider are whether current practice is uncertain, harmful or could be improved and whether the EBG will be helpful for a minority or majority of patients.

Depending on the magnitude of the issue, the EBG may need to focus on areas where there is greatest uncertainty or gaps in the 'know-do'.

Factors to be considered include:

- Prevalence and incidence
- Complexity of and controversy surrounding the condition
- Health economic burden
- Diagnosis rates
- Clearly evident clinical challenges
- Inconsistencies in management
- Benefits for patient outcomes
- Prioritised in policy context
- Prioritised by health professionals
- Prioritised by consumers
- Lack of other evidence based guidance tools

PCOS EBG example

[5] The example is not presented as the gold standard and it is hoped that the practical examples will assist those who are intending to develop or who are developing EBGs. It is important to acknowledge that the example will not apply to all scenarios as there will be variability in the methodology used according to the types of questions and studies that will be considered relevant and acceptable for inclusion in an EBG.

> Currently 70% of Australian women with PCOS remain undiagnosed [5], clinical practice is inconsistent [12], psychological issues are neglected [11] and there is little focus on lifestyle and prevention with most services targeting infertility and costly assisted reproductive technology.

Requirements for Developing an EBG

EBGs are comprehensive and valuable documents with the potential to improve the quality of health care by encouraging interventions of proven benefit and discouraging unnecessary, ineffective or harmful interventions [2] and the requirements for developing a high quality EBG should not be underestimated.

The rigorous nature of their development means that the process can take time and be costly [6]. Therefore one of the first steps is to determine whether you have the capacity, in terms of time, funding, resources and skills, and links with appropriate individuals and groups.

The time and funding required for each stage of EBG is difficult to estimate when the practicalities of each step are not clear. In this chapter we will attempt to outline such practical activities.

While time and funding will vary depending on the people involved and their availability, it is hoped that this chapter will act as a starting point. It may be helpful to contact developers of other high quality guidelines to discuss their experience.

However it is important to keep in mind that it is very difficult to estimate evidence review time as it is dependent on search results, how many studies are identified as relevant as thus the time required to appraise and synthesise each study's characteristics, quality and results.

Clinician and researcher knowledge of the literature will help to estimate how large or small a search yield and subsequent workload is likely to be.

Essential to EBG development is the mix of skills within the team of developers. A useful guideline will benefit from contributors with evidence skills, clinical expertise, consumer perspectives, protected time and access to research evidence. Convening a multidisciplinary EBG development group will be discussed further below.

The Guidelines International Network (G-I-N) facilitates collaboration among EBG developers, researchers, students, stakeholders, implementers and end-users in an effort towards a high standard of EBG development, adaptation, dissemination and implementation; and strive to reduce the duplication of effort by maintaining a resource for data extraction tables called GINDER [Guidelines International Network. [cited 2011 October]; Available from: http://www.g-i-n.net/.] Nevertheless, there is no gold standard methodological framework for developing an effective EBG. Development methodology most helpful to a particular group and topic will depend on the clinical questions, the purpose of the EBG, and the evidence available [5]. However the following guideline development handbooks and tools can be used as guidance on aspects of EBG development and will be referred to in this chapter:

- Centre for Clinical Effectiveness (CCE). Guideline development toolkit [1].
- Scottish Intercollegiate Guideline Network (SIGN). SIGN 50: A guideline developers' handbook [21].
- National Institute for Health and Clinical Excellence (NICE). The Guideline Manual [19].
- National Health and Medical Research Council (NHMRC) Information for Guideline Developers http://www.nhmrc.gov.au/ guidelines/information-guideline-developers [35].
- National Health and Medical Research Council (NHMRC). Procedures and requirements for meeting the 2011 NHMRC standard for clinical practice guidelines [17].
- New Zealand Guidelines Group (NZGG). Handbook for the Preparation of Explicit Evidence-Based Clinical Practice Guidelines [20].
- The AGREE II Instrument. http://www.agreetrust.org/ [32].

Regardless of the method or framework used, whether one or more, the process of every step and the subsequent outcomes should be documented from start to finish.

Reporting of process is what separates EBGs from other types of health information, without which, however rigorous, the user has no way of deciding whether the guidance is trustworthy. The Appraisal of Guidelines for Research and Evaluation Instrument (The AGREE II instrument) provides a framework designed to assess the quality of guidelines, assess the quality of the reporting in guidelines and to inform EBG developers about what should be included in a high quality EBG [32, 33].

Endorsement of EBGs by local, national or international guideline development bodies can help to promote uptake of EBGs by increasing its credibility and sometimes through dissemination.

Some endorsement bodies require developers to follow a particular process which can be arduous and time-intensive and should be accounted for in planning tasks and timelines.

Management of the EBG Development Process

Structure, expertise and skills (clinical and methodological), resources, commitment, leadership and administrative support are essential to the completion of an EBG [1, 5].

Significant input into planning and developing collaborations is critical to a successful process. Also while clinical expertise is important, skills in evidence appraisal, EBG development and project management are vital as is consumer input.

Often guideline development is led by clinicians with a clinical skill set and the importance of these other fundamental skill sets may not be appreciated.

In these cases, attempts at guideline development often falter or even fail to deliver.

Ideally, the process is best managed by one entity that oversees all steps and decision making and ensures that deliverables are met efficiently. Whether this is in the form of an individual or a steering group, or both may depend on the magnitude of the EBG. Above all, organisational, leadership and communication skills are essential to convene a group of EBG developers. In a small EBG, there may be one group that facilitates governance, reporting and development. A larger EBG may require several groups or individuals to ensure the EBG remains on track at an appropriate pace. The PCOS GL is an example of a larger EBG:

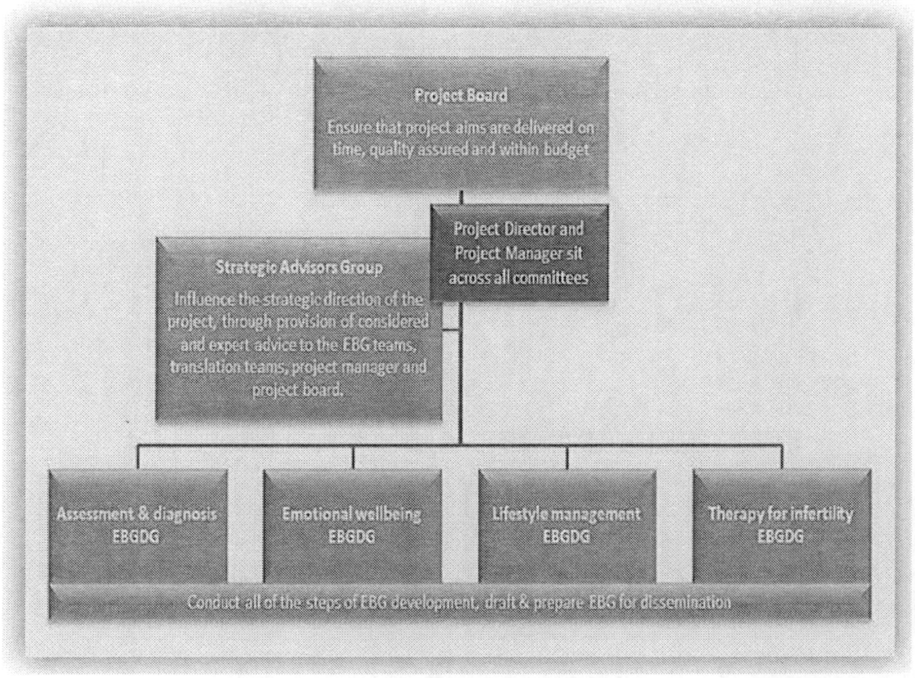

Conflicts of interest should be declared by all involved in developing the guideline. Financial interests in, or close working relationshipswith pharmaceutical companies has the potential to influence the interpretation of evidence from clinicalstudies [21]. While it is not possible to completely eliminate any possible bias from this source, being explicit about the influences on EBG developers makes it possible for readers to assess how likely the guideline recommendations may be based ona biased interpretation of the evidence [21]. This is reiterated in a recent paper by Scott and Guyatt discussing potential solutions to conflicts of interest in developing guidelines [34].

Declaration of interests example templates can be found in:

- Centre for Clinical Effectiveness (CCE). Guideline development toolkit [1].
- Scottish Intercollegiate Guideline Network (SIGN). SIGN 50: A guideline developers' handbook [21].

PCOS EBG Example:

Conflict of interest and confidentiality

Conflict of interest has been proactively managed throughout the guideline development process as outlined in NHMRC standards and procedures for externally developed guidelines [51]. All members of the guideline development groups have provided signed declarations of conflict of interest and a confidentiality agreement. Additionally, declarations of interest were a standing agenda item at each monthly meeting and guideline development group members were requested to detail areas for potential conflict. The process for managing conflict of interest and confidentiality and recorded declarations can be provided on request (jhf.diabetes@monash.edu).

The Steps of EBG Development

Figure 2 outlines the steps of EBG development which will be discussed step by step below.

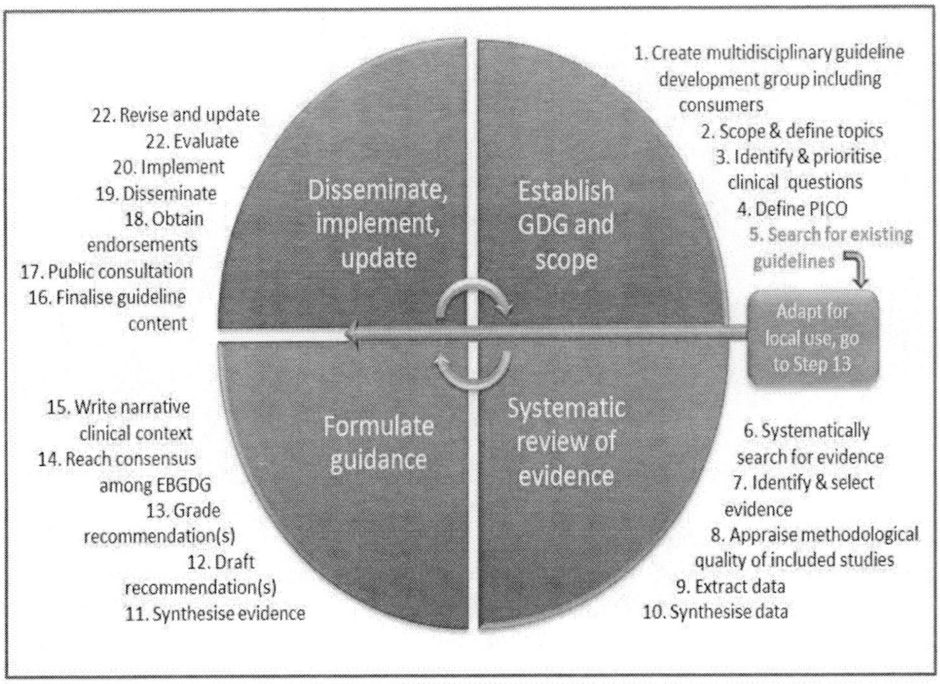

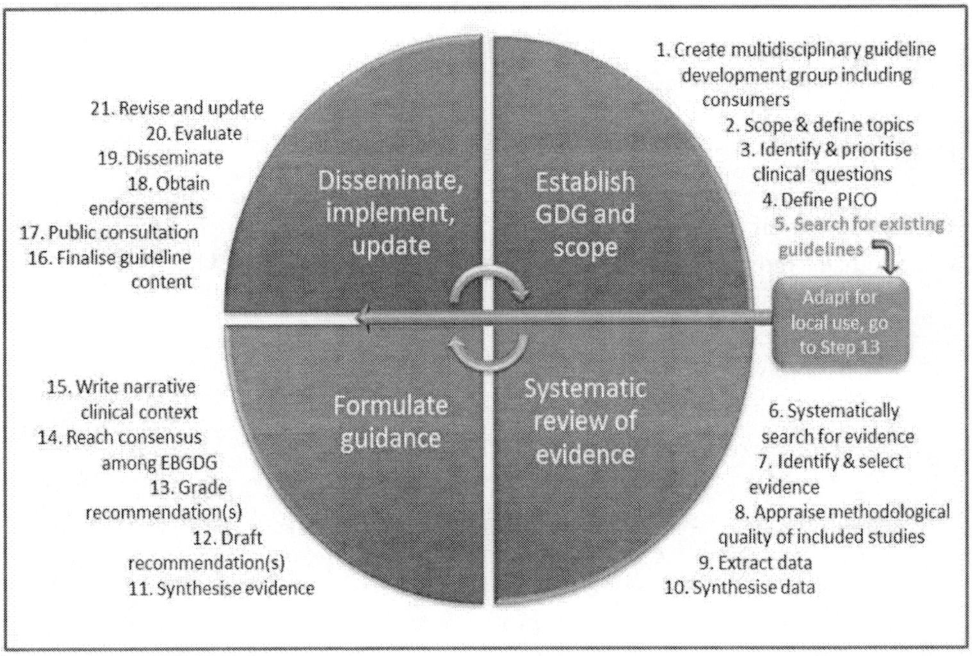

Figure 2. The steps of EBG development.

Establishing and Engaging a Multidisciplinary EBG Development Group

EBG development group (EBGDG) generally refers to the team of individuals who conduct the tasks required to complete an EBG such as drafting the scope; development and prioritisation of clinical questions, conducting the evidence reviews, developing draft recommendations and preparing the guideline for dissemination. Everyone who may use the EBG should be represented in the EBGDG to ensure that the EBG is relevant. This includes representation from any or all of the following: relevant professional groups and societies; clinicians at all levels of seniority with experience in all relevant clinical settings; consumers, carers or consumer representatives; representatives from the Indigenous and culturally and linguistically diverse (CALD) communities (where most relevant); researchers; and evidence review and knowledge translation experts, hence the label multidisciplinary. The benefits of including a wide range of contributors are to gain insight into where there is uncertainty in practice, identifying potential obstacles to EBG implementation [35] and thus what the EBG should address and how dissemination and implementation should be planned. Contributors that are linked with clinical practice, policy and consumer organisations are also invaluable for disseminating the EBG and facilitating change in practice. Practically, the EBGDG should have input from consumers and collective clinical and methodological expertise with capacity to complete the tasks required. It is important to consider the experience and dynamics of the EBGDG members to maximise efficiency for each step of the development process.

PCOS EBG Example:

> Guideline development groups were convened to address each of the four key clinical areas. Expertise was sought through Alliance networks to ensure multidisciplinary participation within each guideline development group. Each guideline development group comprised a chair, professional group members with specific expertise in PCOS and the clinical area of interest (i.e. psychologist in the emotional wellbeing guideline development group), a consumer representative, evidence officers and where possible, a representative to provide context in the Indigenous setting. See Appendix II.

Consumer Participation

The consumer perspective is inevitably different from the clinical or research perspective and will add valuable insight into the scope, content and dissemination plan of the EBG.

Consumers represent the views of the patient which can be overlooked when the EBGDG is focussed on clinical issues [1]. However, it is important to remember that a room of clinicians may be an intimidating environment for a consumer. In order to provide an open and supportive environment for a consumer to be confident to raise and advocate for issues of importance, it may be helpful to recruit more than one consumer representative. Having two consumer representatives means that they can discuss issues together and build confidence before contributing within the EBGDG and if only one can attend a meeting the consumer and patient perspective is still incorporated into EBGDG discussion and decisions [1]. It can also be helpful for the consumer representatives to attend a training course about EBG development [20] with a focus on consensus methods when formulating clinical questions and recommendations.

PCOS EBG Example:

Consumer participation

The peak consumer body in PCOS, Polycystic Ovary Syndrome Association Australia (POSAA) provided consumer representatives who participated in the PCOS Australian Alliance Strategic Advisory Group and the guideline development groups. The President of POSAA is a member of the Project Board and the PCOS Australian Alliance. Consumers have been involved in every stage including formation of the Alliance, proposal to the Department of Health and Ageing for funding, development of the scope, public consultation of the scope and developing and refining the clinical questions and recommendations as part of the guideline development groups. Consumer representatives will also be extensively involved in the translation activities of the guidelines.

Indigenous and CALD Group Participation

To ensure that the EBG is useful for everyone that can benefit, where appropriate, the EBGDG should have representation from consumers who can also provide the perspective of those whose access to care may be different from the general population. There is little practical guidance to assist with the most appropriate methods to engage Indigenous and CALD communities; however common sense and respect for cultural differences should prevail.

PCOS EBG Example

Indigenous representation

Indigenous representation was present on the PCOS Australian Alliance Strategic Advisory Group (a member of the Australian Indigenous Doctors Association) and the guideline development groups comprised clinicians with experience working with Indigenous communities. The Programme Manager for the Jean Hailes Foundation for Women's Health National Indigenous Women's Health Programme provided oversight for Indigenous issues and considerations across all recommendations in the guideline.

Engagement

EBGDG members need to be *engaged* for an EBG to be high quality and useful.This may mean contributing in group discussion settings, either in a brainstorming capacity or by contributing to high level discussion based on pre-reading; or by written contribution.

It is very helpful if EBGDG members are engaged and ready to hit the ground running from the beginning, particularly for tasks such as proposing the scope and proposing and prioritising clinical questions, as these steer the content of the EBG and should not be altered once the evidence review stage has begun. Maintaining engagement can be tricky and is essential to efficiency, particularly in the evidence review stage where quick decisions and responses are required by evidence reviewers who may not have the clinical expertise to move forward on practical tasks such as deciding whether a study is relevant due to inconsistency in terminology or synthesising complicated clinical data. Thorough planning of selection criteria to attempt avoiding this will be discussed later. Where meetings are scheduled according to deliverables, missing a meeting may delay a deliverable by a month and if key contributors are missing for multiple meetings, this may have a major impact on timelines [1]. Having said this, it is important that terms of reference [1], including expectations (of individuals and groups) and timelines, are outlined and agreed upon at the very beginning and that steps are taken to minimise any deviation, particularly given that clinicians and consumers often have competing priorities and their participation in EBGDGs is usually in a voluntary, unpaid capacity. Terms of reference should include specific objectives and deliverables with respect to expected contribution; as well as frequency and length of meetings.

Training

EBGDG members may need support and training to ensure in-depth knowledge of the EBG development process and an understanding of the requirements for carrying out each members' role effectively [19]. An understanding by the EBG member of how their role fits within the overall process has the potential to encourage efficient and effective contribution.

PCOS EBG Example:

The chairs of each guideline development group attended a one day workshop, facilitated by the Jean Hailes Foundation for Women's Health and the Centre for Clinical Effectiveness, where the methods of reviewing evidence and guideline development were described in detail. The purpose of this workshop was to familiarise the chairs with:

- the process of guideline development overall
- the process of identifying, appraising and synthesising evidence in a format to facilitate the formulation of evidence-based recommendations
- grading the strength of evidence and its suitability to support evidence-based recommendations
- when to facilitate discussion and clinical judgement to formulate clinical consensus recommendations in the absence of evidence

At this workshop the chairs also participated in an exercise to generate potential clinical questions.

In addition, at the beginning of the first guideline development group monthly meeting, the evidence advisor briefly described the processes for evidence-based guideline development and these processes were reiterated as the evidence reviews were presented each month.

For more guidance on establishing a multidisciplinary EBGDG, refer to:

- Centre for Clinical Effectiveness (CCE). Guideline Development Toolkit [1].
- National Institute for Health and Clinical Excellence (NICE).The Guideline Manual [19].
- New Zealand Guidelines Group (NZGG). Handbook for the Preparation of Explicit Evidence-based Clinical Practice Guidelines [20].

1. Defining Scope and Clinical Topics

Once the topic for the EBG has been decided, a scope should be prepared. The scope forms the basis of the EBG and provides a snapshot of its content and usability. It should include description of the topic and the context in which the EBG should be read. The target users and target patients should be clearly specified. Scoping the EBG is the fundamental step that sets the direction for all that follows and helps to estimate the time and resources needed. Scope may be decided by the composition of the EBGDG or conversely the scope may influence the composition of the EBGDG. At this stage ensure that the development of the EBG is manageable by confining the focus on areas of greatest need and make every effort to remain within the scope. It is important to reach agreement among all EBG committees on the scope before commencing development. Extending the scope (scope creep) during the development process not only has the potential to introduce bias, but also to increase workload and blow out timelines. An example EBG scope that includes clinical need, purpose, patient population, setting and audience and topics can be found in the *Evidence-based guideline for the assessment and management of polycystic ovary syndrome* at http://www.managingpcos.org.au/pcos-evidence-based-guidelines. For more guidance on preparing a scope, refer to *The Guideline Manual* by NICE [19].

2. Identify and Prioritise Clinical Questions

"Although it is not always recognised, each interaction between a clinician and a patient/consumer generates several clinical questions." [20]. This is the first and most important step in EBG development and the first on the road to developing a search strategy, selecting studies, critical appraisal and data collection. When creating a list of clinical questions, it is helpful to think practically through the patient journey. Consulting widely will help to ensure that the clinical questions in the EBG are useful.

PCOS EBG Example:

Development and prioritisation of the clinical questions addressed in this guideline was conducted in three stages. First, in the workshop described above, attended by the chairs of each clinical area and the evidence officers, clinical questions were generated. Secondly, the clinical questions were distributed to all members of each corresponding guideline development group, the Project Board and the PCOS Australian Alliance Strategic Advisory Group. All members were invited to provide feedback on the suitability of the existing questions and to suggest additional clinical questions, if appropriate. Thirdly, the clinical questions were consolidated and distributed once again to guideline development group members who were asked to prioritise each question according to a ranking of 1-6. Rankings were compiled and 22 highly relevant and important clinical questions were agreed and form this guideline.

While there may be an abundance of interesting evidence available, unless it is answering a question that clinicians, policy makers or consumers are asking it may not worthwhile pursuing [20]. Given the time and resource limitations of EBG development, the number of questions should be kept manageable.

Manageable is defined by the available time and resources. Questions should always be assessed for priority, where practice is uncertain or unknown; and if a question doesn't make the a priori list, then it doesn't make the guideline. Introducing clinical questions after development has begun has the potential to introduce bias and increases the risk of missing timelines. Review questions must be well defined, the process for which is discussed below.

3. Define Clinical Questions and Translate into Selection Criteria Using PICO

The selection (inclusion and exclusion) criteria, used for selecting the research evidence that will be used to answer the question, must be decided a priori for each clinical question. The structure of the question and subsequent selection criteria will depend on whether the question is about prevention or therapy, diagnosis, prognosis or aetiology. There are various frameworks for exploring these types of questions. The PICO framework focusses on the Population of interest, Intervention (whether in the form of a treatment, cause or prognostic factor), Comparison and Outcomes. The PECOT framework, used by the NZGG, focusses on Population, Exposure, Comparison, Outcome and Time [20]. These frameworks help to define the detail within each question and to set the a priori criteria for searching, including and excluding studies, synthesising evidence and drafting recommendations. Inclusion of detail at this stage is also helpful for the evidence review team, who may not have the clinical expertise to decipher the myriad of definitions, variable terminology and outcome scales and ranges. Criteria should be specific and comprehensive and not limited to those listed here, that are simply provided as a starting point.

For the population in the clinical question, detail should include information such as age, gender, setting, co-morbidities, previous or current medication; the intervention or group of interventions should specify type, dose, frequency; the comparison should be specified as no intervention, another intervention (including detail about type, dose, frequency), usual care, wait list; relevant measurable outcomes to be able to answer your question should be listed with corresponding acceptable scales and ranges. Below is an example from the PCOS EBG for the clinical question: In women with PCOS is ovarian surgery, compared to nothing, placebo or other infertility treatment, effective for improving fertility outcomes?

Study selection criteria

Patient	**Inclusion:** Women of any age, ethnicity and weight with PCOS diagnosed by Rotterdam, NIH or AIS AND 1) at least one patent tube 2) normal sperm AND 3) have never been treated or been exposed to treatment for infertility (therapy naïve) OR 4) have been treated or exposed to treatment OR 5) have been treated or exposed to clomiphene citrate and ovulate but don't conceive (clomid failure) OR 6) have been treated or exposed to clomid and don't ovulate (clomid resistant). **Exclusion:** Women without diagnosis of PCOS.		
Intervention	**Inclusion:** Any type of ovarian surgery, including: laser or diathermy laparoscopy, laparotomy, transvaginal hydro-laparoscopy. **Exclusion:** Placebo, no intervention or any intervention other than a type of ovarian surgery.		
Comparison	**Inclusion:** Placebo, no intervention, other infertility treatment interventions including metformin, clomid, aromatase inhibitors, gonadotrophin, or ovarian surgery in combination with other infertility treatment intervention(s). **Exclusion:** Any type of ovarian surgery alone.		
Outcomes	**Inclusion:** Live birth rate, pregnancy rate (biochemical or clinical ultrasound), ovulation, single and multiple pregnancies, miscarriage rate, other adverse events, quality of life, cost effectiveness. **Exclusion:** None.		
Study type	**Inclusion:** Systematic reviews and RCTs addressing the outcomes are sought. **Exclusion:** Any study lower than an RCT.	**Publication Date**	Any

For more guidance on defining clinical questions and selection criteria, refer to:

- National Institute for Health and Clinical Excellence (NICE).The Guideline Manual [19].
- New Zealand Guidelines Group (NZGG). Handbook for the Preparation of Explicit Evidence-based Clinical Practice Guidelines [20].

4. Establish Need for New or Adapted Guidelines

Given the time and resource-intensive nature of EBG development, a search for existing high quality EBGs should be conducted before starting a new one. Adaptation of an EBG to a local context, when facilitated by key local knowledge translation experts who have experience in applying evidence to a local setting, has the potential to lead to better uptake of the EBG and its recommendations and ensure sustainable quality of care [6].

Search and identify existing EBGs

Like development of EBGs, adaptation should follow a systematic and transparent process from the search and identification stage to how their recommendations are used. Below is the systematic search used to identify existing EBGs in the PCOS EBG.

Internet searches to identify relevant websites

The reviewers were aware of websites of guideline clearinghouses, guideline developers, centres of evidence-based practice, Australian government health services and websites of specific relevance known to contain evidence-based resources. Additional websites of specific relevance were sought via an internet search using the Google 'Advanced Search' function with the following string:

(((polycystic AND (ovary OR ovarian)) AND (disease OR syndrome)) OR PCOS OR PCOD) AND (professional OR association OR organisation OR organization OR college OR society OR academy OR peak)

Website searches to identify relevant evidence-based guidelines

Where an internal search engine was available, websites were searched. If no search engine was available, lists of guidelines, publications or other resources identified on the site were scanned for relevant documents.

Internet searches to identify relevant evidence-based guidelines and systematic reviews

An internet search strategy was conducted to identify evidence-based guidelines and systematic reviews using the Google 'Advanced Search' function with the following string:

(((polycystic AND (ovary OR ovarian)) AND (disease OR syndrome)) OR PCOS OR PCOD) AND (guideline OR evidence OR systematic)

Adapting an existing EBG

We will not detail the process of adaption as we are focusing on de novo development of EBGs here, but do encourage the reader to seek the resources mentioned below for further detail.

Stakeholders including consumers should be involved at each step of adaptation and factors that influence and inform recommendations, including those in the original EBG should be reported, along with reasons for any modifications to the original guideline [36]. Steps, often lacking in EBGs, that can be addressed in the adaptation process include: piloting of the EBG among target users, consumer input and review, external review, consideration of organisational barriers, cost implications and updating plans [6].

Adaptation of EBGs is addressed in varying levels of detail in handbooks for preparing guidelines from the Council of Europe, the National Health and Medical Research Council (NHMRC, Australia), the National Institute for Clinical Excellence (NICE, UK), the New Zealand Guidelines Group (NZGG) and the Scottish Intercollegiate Guidelines Network (SIGN) [4]. The ADAPTE framework manual and tools is based upon evidence based and rigorous development principles and is the gold standard for determining whether a guideline is suitable for adaptation and introduces concepts for adapting guidelines from their original setting to different contexts, whether cultural or organisational, using a step-by-step process [37].

The existing EBG should provide enough information to decide if it fits the PICO and selection criteria, which should be as close as possible, so that time unpicking the evidence is minimised ie. if you only want evidence at or higher than the level of randomised controlled trials (RCTs), you will need to think carefully about whether you adapt an EBG that has synthesised evidence from non-RCTs.

In some instances, you may need to contact the EBG developers for a copy of their clinical questions, PICO and inclusion criteria and sometimes their evidence tables if they are not detailed in the EBG that is accessible.

Without this level of detail there is a risk of finding the EBGDG half way through the Adapte process before realising that the evidence is not of sufficient quality and that time could have been better spent starting a new evidence review to answer the clinical question.

Evidence Review

The evidence review stage is the systematic identification, appraisal and synthesis of available evidence to answer a clinical question and subsequently formulate recommendations. Every evidence review should begin with the preparation of a protocol that includes the PICO selection criteria and the plan for conducting the search for evidence as well as a priori criteria for appraising the quality and extracting outcome data from the identified studies. A plan for how the data will be synthesised (ie. meta-analysis), should it be appropriate, should also be addressed in the protocol. Protocols may have elements that are consistent across all clinical questions and elements that are specific to individual clinical questions. For more guidance on preparing an evidence review protocol, refer to *Systematic reviews: CRD's guidance for undertaking reviews in health care* by the Centre for Reviews and Dissemination [38].

1. Systematically Search for Evidence

A systematic search strategy should be designed to identify the best available evidence to answer each of the clinical questions. A search strategy includes the sources that will be searched and the terms and limits (eg. year, language, study type) used to search those sources. While the same sources should be used for all questions, the terms and combinations of terms may be different for each question. The exception to the rule of using the same sources may be found in a broad EBG that covers different topics warranting the search of different additional topic specific databases such as PsycInfo for an emotional wellbeing question as well as PEDro for a physiotherapy related question. The important point is that a consistently comprehensive search strategy is used and reported across an EBG according to the a priori protocol. Searches should be documented so that they are reproducible [19].

Databases

SIGN requires that a search strategy cover at least *The Cochrane Library*, Medline, Embase and the internet, and in most cases should cover sources specific to the topic as well as those that cover health economics literature [21]. Studies with less 'trendy' findings may not be published in the major sources but may still answer the clinical question and be of sufficient quality to include in the evidence review. Therefore, if time and resources permit, it may be of benefit to hand-search particularly relevant journals not listed in the major databases as well as grey literature such as unpublished reports and reference lists of included studies.

PCOS EBG Example:

The following electronic databases were employed to identify relevant literature:

- Australasian Medical Index
- CINAHL
- The Cochrane Library
- Cochrane Database of Systematic Reviews (Cochrane Reviews)
- Database of Abstracts of Reviews of Effects (Other Reviews)
- Cochrane Central Register of Controlled Trials (Clinical Trials)
- Cochrane Database of Methodology Reviews (Methods Reviews)
- The Cochrane Methodology Register (Methods Studies)
- Health Technology Assessment Database (Technology Assessments)
- NHS Economic Evaluation Database (Economic Evaluations)
- EMBASE
- EBM Reviews (OVID)
- Medline (OVID)
- Medline in-process and other non-indexed citations (OVID)
- PsycInfo (OVID)

Search Terms

The terms used in the search should be based on the selection criteria for each clinical question. Expand the list of selection criteria with any alternative terms including alternate spellings and variant word endings for each of the criteria. The idea is to create search strings of the terms to describe each of the components of the selection criteria (PICO) and then combine them using the various tools available to search for relevant articles efficiently, see the example below for a search string for the 'P' component. If required, outcomes can be used in the search string, however if the search yield is low, it may not be necessary to limit the search further.

Controlled vocabularies

Medical subject headings (MeSH), used in Medline, are updated by the United States National Library of Medicine (NLM) and are a comprehensive controlled vocabulary arranged in a tree structure to index journal articles and books and serves as a thesaurus to use when searching [39]. When MeSH are used in a search, all articles within the Medline database that are indexed (coded) to the MeSH heading will be retrieved. As demonstrated in the PCOS EBG example, in search term number one 'exp polycystic ovary syndrome/', 'polycystic ovary syndrome' is the MeSH and the 'exp' preceding the MeSH indicates that all articles indexed to 'polycystic ovary syndrome' *and* all the subheadings below it in the tree will be retrieved. Alternatively if the 'exp' is not used, as demonstrated in search term number six 'anovulation/' in the PCOS EBG example below, articles indexed to the MeSH will be retrieved, but articles indexed to a subheading lower in the tree will not be retrieved. For more detailed guidance on this form of searching, refer to the MeSH section on the NLM website [39]. While this is an efficient method to search, it is estimated that 50% of articles in Medline are inadequately or incorrectly classified by subheading [40], therefore text words should be combined with MeSH in a search string to ensure that all relevant articles are retrieved.

Similar controlled vocabularies can be found in other databases such as Embase and CINAHL.

Text Words

Keeping with the 'P' component of the search, add each of the population terms as text words. This means that the search will retrieve all articles that contain the text word wherever you specify ie. in the title, abstract or subject heading. In the example below, the '.mp', which stands for 'multi-purpose' has been used at the end of text words to retrieve all articles containing the text word in their title, original title, abstract, subject heading, name of substance, and registry word fields.

Truncation

Truncation symbols will depend on the database being searched. The symbols '$' and '*' are most commonly used to truncate text words to allow for different word endings or spellings. For example 'polycystic ovar$.mp.' will retrieve articles that use the terms: polycystic ovary, polycystic ovaries and polycystic ovarian.

Boolean Operators

Boolean operators can be used to connect the terms together in the search string, whether to increase or restrict the search. Using 'OR' will increase the results of the search by being inclusive of all articles that contain *any* of the terms that are connected with an 'OR'. Using the PCOS EBG example below, an article that contains any of the terms from 1-10 will be retrieved by the search. Using 'AND' limits the search to articles that contain *all* of the terms that are connected with an 'AND'. For example if search term one was combined with the term 'laparoscopic ovarian surgery', the search would only retrieve articles that included both 'polycystic ovary syndrome' *and* 'laparoscopic ovarian surgery'.

PCOS EBG Example:

Search terms in Medline*	
1	exp polycystic ovary syndrome/
2	polycystic ovar$.mp.
3	poly-cystic ovar$.mp.
4	PCO$.mp.
5	(stein-leventhal or leventhal).mp.
6	anovulation/
7	anovulat$.mp.
8	oligo-ovulat$.mp.
9	oligoovulat$.mp.
10	(ovar$ adj5 (sclerocystic or polycystic or poly-cystic or degenerat$ or hyperandrogen$ or hyper-ndrogen$)).mp.
11	or/1 - 10

For detailed instructions on how to use the different searching tools and to save search strings, you can contact a reference librarian or refer to:

- New Zealand Guidelines Group (NZGG). Handbook for the Preparation of Explicit Evidence-based Clinical Practice Guidelines [20].
- Online Help Centre in NLM [39].
- Systematic reviews: CRD's guidance for undertaking reviews in health care by Centre for Reviews and Dissemination [38].

2. Identification and Selection of Evidence

When large numbers of articles are retrieved, a reference manager (eg. Endnote) may be helpful to manage the process of identifying (also known as screening) articles for inclusion. Articles can be exported to the reference manager and the help centres in each of the searching databases provide instructions on how to do this. Use the selection criteria to screen each article and decide whether it is relevant to answering the clinical question. Some articles may be excluded after reading (and therefore based on) an obvious title, others may be excluded only after reading the abstract and some articles may need to be retrieved in full text before they can be assessed. The PRISMA flow diagram can be used for this stage as it maps out the number of records identified, included and excluded, and the reasons for exclusions [41].

PCOS EBG Example:

Studies were selected and appraised by one reviewer in consultation with colleagues using study selection and appraisal criteria established *a priori*. A broad search was conducted to capture all studies relevant to the guideline: therapy for infertility in women with PCOS. An initial search returned 4108 articles of which 2047 duplicates were removed, leaving 2061 articles for review. Of these, 56 articles were relevant to ovarian surgery. The articles were reviewed by title and abstract. When a decision could not be made based on title and abstract alone, full text was retrieved. Fifty full text articles were retrieved for review and **four articles met the inclusion and exclusion criteria.**

3. Quality Appraisal of Evidence

"Ultimately, quality assessment helps answer the question of whether the studies are robust enough to guide treatment, prevention, diagnostic or policy decisions."[38]. Critical appraisal of the evidence explores the strengths and weaknesses of the included studies and whether they are susceptible to the different types of bias. Risk of bias assessment frameworks are based on the types of bias that are influenced by aspects of study design which may have an effect on the trustworthiness of the study's results. These frameworks usually differ between study designs. Where EBG development is aligned with a guideline organisation or endorsing body (eg. NHMRC, NICE, SIGN) there may be a prescribed framework. Otherwise, use appraisal criteria that address the types of bias to systematically decide upon the likely direction of bias in each study. A critical appraisal framework for a RCT may include components such as whether conflicts of interest were declared by the study authors; selection criteria for inclusion of participants was reported adequately; adequate methods of randomisation, allocation of participants to groups and blinding was reported; outcomes were adequately measured and reported; powering and statistics were performed appropriately; and whether data are reported and analysed appropriately.

Cohort, case control and case series study appraisal frameworks will focus on selection, similarity and appropriate representation of groups and their exposure instead of randomisation and allocation concealment. For more detail about critical appraisal and suggested frameworks, refer to the following:

- Centre for Clinical Effectiveness (CCE). Critical Appraisal Templates by CCE [42].
- Systematic reviews: CRD's guidance for undertaking reviews in health care by Centre for Reviews and Dissemination [38].
- Scottish Intercollegiate Guideline Network (SIGN). SIGN 50: A guideline developers' handbook [21].
- New Zealand Guidelines Group (NZGG). Handbook for the Preparation of Explicit Evidence-based Clinical Practice Guidelines [20].
- National Institute for Health and Clinical Excellence (NICE). The Guideline Manual [19].
- Cochrane Handbook for Systematic Reviews of Interventions www.cochrane.org /resources/handbook/[Higgins J., Green S. Cochrane Handbook for Systematic Reviews of Interventions. Version 5.1.0 [updated March 2011]: The Cochrane Collaboration; 2011.]

The PCOS EBG example below employs the CCE framework for assessing risk of bias.

Methodological quality of the included studies was assessed using criteria developed *a priori* according to study design (i.e. quality appraisal criteria used for an RCT is different to that used for a cohort study) [52]. Individual quality items were investigated using a descriptive component approach. Any disagreement or uncertainty was resolved by discussion among the guideline development team to reach a consensus. Using this approach, each study was allocated a risk of bias rating (see Table 2). Quality appraisal and data extraction tables for each evidence review can be found in the supporting document titled 'Evidence report', which can be found at www.managingpcos.org.au/pcos-evidence-based-guidelines.

Table 2. Risk of bias ratings [52]

Rating	Description
Low	All of the criteria have been fulfilled or where criteria have not been fulfilled it is very unlikely the conclusions of the study would be affected.
Moderate	Some of the criteria have been fulfilled and those criteria that have not been fulfilled may affect the conclusions of the study.
High	Few or no criteria fulfilled or the conclusions of the study are likely or very likely to be affected.
Insufficient information	Not enough information provided on methodological quality to be able to determine risk of bias.

4. Data Extraction

The process of data extraction is about systematically recording the results of the included studies according to a priori defined outcomes. Below is an example of the types of information about study characteristics and results that may be extracted. Extracting data for outcomes that were not planned a priori in the protocol has the potential to introduce bias and should be avoided.

PCOS EBG Example:

Data, according to the selection criteria, was extracted from included studies using a specially developed data extraction form [52]. Information was collected on general details (title, authors, reference/source, country, year of publication, setting), participants (age, sex, inclusion/exclusion criteria, withdrawals/losses to follow-up, subgroups), results (point estimates and measures of variability, frequency counts for dichotomous variables, number of participants, intention-to-treat analysis) and validity results. Quality appraisal and data extraction tables for each evidence review can be found in the supporting document titled 'Evidence report', which can be found at www.managingpcos.org.au/pcos-evidence-based-guidelines.

For more detail about data extraction, types of data and suggested templates, refer to the following:

- Centre for Clinical Effectiveness (CCE). Critical Appraisal Templates [42].
- Systematic reviews: CRD's guidance for undertaking reviews in health care by Centre for Reviews and Dissemination [38].
- Scottish Intercollegiate Guideline Network (SIGN). SIGN 50: A guideline developers' handbook [21].

- New Zealand Guidelines Group (NZGG). Handbook for the Preparation of Explicit Evidence-based Clinical Practice Guidelines [20].
- National Institute for Health and Clinical Excellence (NICE). The Guideline Manual [19].

5. Data Synthesis

In order to make a summary statement about the effect of the intervention, data may be summarised, by presenting the findings narratively in tables or discussion text; or quantitatively, using statistical methods such as meta-analyses. A meta-analysis is a statistical technique for combining (pooling) the results of a number of studies that address thesame question and report on the same outcomes to produce a summary result. Where it is appropriate to perform meta-analysis, the aim is to derivemore precise and clear information from a large data pool.

It is generally more reliably likely to confirmor refute a hypothesis than the individual trials.

It is outside the scope of this chapter to provide specific guidance on when and how to use the numerous different types of data and methods of data syntheses; however detailed guidance can be found in the following:

- Systematic reviews: CRD's guidance for undertaking reviews in health care by Centre for Reviews and Dissemination [38]/
- Cochrane Handbook for Systematic Reviews of Interventions www.cochrane.org /resources/handbook/. [Higgins J, Green S. Cochrane Handbook for Systematic Reviews of Interventions. Version 5.1.0 [updated March 2011]: The Cochrane Collaboration; 2011.]

6. Evidence Synthesis

Summaries of Individual Studies

A summary of each study, in terms of its characteristics, risk of bias and findings is helpful and may be as simple as a few points at the end of the study appraisal and data extraction. In addition, some national and guideline development bodies have classifications for individual studies. For example the NHMRC in Australia classifies studies by ‘levels of evidence’ as well as a quality rating and the levels are assigned according to the type of study (eg. intervention, diagnostic accuracy, prognosis, aetiology, screening). Below is an example of the NHMRC levels assigned to intervention-type studies [43].

Level	Intervention studies
I	A systematic review of level II studies
II	A randomised controlled trial
III-1	A pseudo-randomised controlled trial (i.e. alternate allocation or some other method)
III-2	A comparative study with concurrent controls: ■ Non-randomised, experimental trial ■ Cohort study ■ Case-control study ■ Interrupted time series with a control group
III-3	A comparative study without concurrent controls: ■ Historical control study ■ Two or more single arm studies ■ Interrupted time series without a parallel control group
IV	Case series with either post-test or pre-test/post-test outcomes

Levels of evidence are defined slightly differently according to the guideline development body, these can be found at:

- National Health and Medical Research Council (NHMRC). Procedures and requirements for meeting the 2011 NHMRC standard for clinical practice guidelines [17].
- Scottish Intercollegiate Guideline Network (SIGN). SIGN 50: A guideline developers' handbook [21].
- New Zealand Guidelines Group (NZGG). Handbook for the Preparation of Explicit Evidence-based Clinical Practice Guidelines [20].
- National Institute for Health and Clinical Excellence (NICE). The Guideline Manual [19].

Summaries of the Body of Evidence

All of the studies that answer a particular clinical question, known as the body of evidence, should be summarised together; and the approach for doing this should be consistent across all clinical questions. Some guideline development bodies prescribe what should be discussed and how it should be presented.

Independent EBG developers should ensure that similarities and differences between studies are discussed with a focus on risk of bias and consistency in population groups, interventions and findings.

This discussion will be the link between the evidence and the recommendations of the EBG and the quality and consistency of the evidence will help to decide how much emphasis should be placed on each recommendation through the use of grading frameworks.

This will be explored further below.

7. Drafting Recommendations

When drafting recommendations, it is important to think about care alternatives to provide options for shared decision making between the patient and the health professional [2].

Recommendations should be clear and unambiguous and provide action oriented guidance [1] in answer to each clinical question.

The language used should be consistent and reflect practical judgment and a balance of benefits and harms.

PCOS EBG Example:

> The words "should", "could" and "should not" do not directly reflect the grade or classification allocated to a recommendation and are independent descriptors intended to reflect the judgment of the multidisciplinary guideline development group on the practical application of the recommendation, balancing benefits and harms. Where the word "should" is used in the recommendations, the guideline development group judged that the benefits of the recommendation (whether evidence-based or clinical consensus) clearly exceed the harms, and that the recommendation can be trusted to guide practice. Where the word "could" is used, either the quality of evidence was underpowered, or the available studies demonstrated little clear advantage of one approach over another, or the balance of benefits to harm was unclear. Where the words "should not" are used, there is either a lack of appropriate evidence, or the harms outweigh the benefits.

Evidence Based Recommendations

Evidence based recommendations are drafted based on the findings of the body of evidence for each clinical question where it is available and should consider the clinical and consumer perspectives to ensure that the recommendation is relevant, as well as reliable. Even with strong, high quality evidence available, recommendations should incorporate value judgments, balancing benefits, harms and patient preference [2].

Where recommendations are based on evidence, a specific explanation about the link between the evidence and recommendation must be provided. If, after EBGDG discussion, the recommendation is substantially different from the findings of the body of evidence, a very strong justification will need to be proposed. This may arise, for example, on the basis of relative cost or treatment availability [1]. Using the PCOS EBG as an example, to answer the question "In women with PCOS, is clomiphene citrate, compared to placebo, no treatment or another intervention, effective for improving fertility outcomes?" the body of evidence found that clomiphene citrate was statistically better than placebo for fertility outcomes and the EBGDG knew of additional implementation considerations, therefore the evidence based recommendation and practice point (discussed further below) are as follows:

Recommendations

Evidence-based recommendation		
7.1a	Clomiphene citrate should be first line pharmacological therapy to improve fertility outcomes in women with polycystic ovary syndrome and anovulatory infertility, with no other infertility factors.	A
Clinical practice point		
7.1b	The risk of multiple pregnancy is increased with clomiphene citrate use and therefore monitoring is recommended.	

Consensus Recommendations

High quality primary research to inform recommendations is often lacking and the evidence that is available is frequently misleading, mostly due to poor study design [2]. Thereforein the absence of sufficient quality evidence, consensus recommendations can be made using considered judgment, based on clinical expertise and consumer perspective. Formulation of consensus recommendations will be discussed further below. Practice points alongside recommendations may be helpful tips on how to safely and effectively implement the recommendation, but it is important that these are recognisable as statements arising from EBGDG discussion, and where evidence has not been sought.

PCOS EBG Example:

> Where there was insufficient or no evidence to make an evidence-based recommendation, a clinical consensus or research recommendation was made based on the clinical expertise of the multidisciplinary guideline development group. Where important issues arose from discussion of evidence-based or clinical consensus recommendations, and thus evidence was not sought, clinical practice points have been provided. They are essential tips on how to safely and effectively implement the recommendations.

Using the PCOS EBG as an example, there was insufficient evidence to answer the question "In adolescents, what are the most effective criteria to diagnose polycystic ovaries on ultrasound?" therefore using the expertise of the EBGDG, the recommendation and practice point are as follows:

Recommendations

Clinical consensus recommendation	
1.3a	Given the apparent lack of specificity of polycystic ovaries on ultrasound in adolescents, generally, ultrasound should not be recommended first line in this age group for diagnosis of polycystic ovary syndrome pending further research. If pelvic ultrasounds are to be ordered in adolescents, the results should be interpreted with caution.
Clinical practice point	
1.3b	Vaginal ultrasound is not appropriate in adolescents who have not been sexually active.

It is essential that all recommendations are clearly labelled so that the reader can identify the different types of recommendations, how they were derived and how much importance should be placed on each.

Recommendations should be accompanied by a discussion about the importance of the recommendation and the impact of the recommendation on clinical practice as well as organisational issues that may affect their uptake and implementation. This should include how they fit with current guidance, particularly where there is overlap across broad guidelines covering similar topics.

PCOS EBG Example:

> Each recommendation is supported by a discussion (in the chapters of this document) about the clinical need for the question, the body of evidence identified to answer the question and the clinical impact of the resulting recommendation(s), including potential changes in usual care and the way care is organised, organisational barriers and resource implications. Such organisational issues are difficult to quantify without conducting methodologically rigorous assessments of relevant services and resources, therefore the clinical experience of the multidisciplinary guideline development groups was drawn upon for these discussions.

Examples of formulating recommendations from the evidence can be found in the *Evidence-based guideline for the assessment and management of polycystic ovary syndrome: evidence report* at http://www.managingpcos.org.au/pcos-evidence-based-guidelines. Specific guidance according to guideline development bodies can be found at:

- National Health and Medical Research Council (NHMRC). Procedures and requirements for meeting the 2011 NHMRC standard for clinical practice guidelines [17]
- National Health and Medical Research Council (NHMRC). Additional levels of evidence and grades for recommendations for developers of guidelines [43]
- Scottish Intercollegiate Guideline Network (SIGN). SIGN 50: A guideline developers' handbook [21].
- New Zealand Guidelines Group (NZGG). Handbook for the Preparation of Explicit Evidence-based Clinical Practice Guidelines [20].
- National Institute for Health and Clinical Excellence (NICE). The Guideline Manual [19].

8. Grading Evidence Based Recommendations

Guideline recommendations are graded to differentiate between those based on strong evidence and those based on weak evidence [21] and to help stratify the recommendations and decide where the recommendations fit in the overall care pathway.

The overall grade should also reflect the strength of the recommendation in terms of trust or confidence practitioners can have in the recommendation when applied in a clinical situation.

The NHMRC approach assigns a grade to each evidence based recommendation using a body of evidence matrix, where an individual component grade is assigned for each of the following according to the body of evidence:

- Volume of evidence – assigned based on the number of studies and the methodological quality of the studies in the body of evidence.
- Consistency of the evidence – assigned based on the similarity in characteristics of the population and study design; and agreement between the studies in the body of evidence.
- Clinical impact of the recommendation – assigned based on the degree of clinical impact, which may depend on current practice and organisational implications.
- Generalisability - assigned based on the generalizability of the body of evidence to the EBG patient population and setting.
- Applicability – assigned based on the applicability of the body of evidence to the Australian healthcare context.

Each individual component is assigned a grade of A-D, where A represents 'excellent', B is 'good', C is 'satisfactory' and D is 'poor' [43].

These are compiled to reach an overall 'grade' of A-D, where an A or B can only be assigned if the individual components for volume and consistency are both graded A or B [43].

Grading the evidence informing each recommendation can also aid the consensus process and can provide the opportunity to prompt and to document any discussion about alignment with or deviation from the evidence; agreement and disagreement among EBGDG members; or unresolved issues when finalising and grading each recommendation.

PCOS EBG Example:

Table 4. The strength of the recommendations can be identified throughout the guideline with the following grades (from NHMRC levels of evidence and grades for recommendations for developers of guidelines [14]):

Grade	Description
A	Body of evidence can be trusted to guide practice.
B	Body of evidence can be trusted to guide practice in most situations.
C	Body of evidence provides some support for recommendation but care should be taken in its application.
D	Body of evidence is weak and recommendation must be applied with caution.

Table 5. Classifications of recommendations for which a Grade cannot be applied.

Classification	Description
CR	In the absence of evidence, a clinical consensus recommendation is made by the guideline development group.
PP	Evidence not sought. A practice point is made by the guideline development group where important issues arose from discussion of evidence-based or clinical consensus recommendations.

For more detail about the NHMRC approach and other approaches to grading the evidence and evidence based recommendations, refer to:

- National Health and Medical Research Council (NHMRC). Additional levels of evidence and grades for recommendations for developers of guidelines by NHMRC [43].
- The GRADE approach by the Grade Working Group [44].
- Scottish Intercollegiate Guideline Network (SIGN). SIGN 50: A guideline developers' handbook [21].

9. Reaching Consensus on Recommendations

Whether consensus needs to be reached on analready drafted evidence based recommendation or needs to be reached to develop a recommendation in the absence of evidence, it is imperative that the approach used is described and that each step of the process is documented.

It must be clear to those who were not involved in the decision making process how EBG developers were able to arrive at their recommendations [21].

Consensus approaches include informal discussion or formal methods such as the nominal group technique, the Delphi technique or consensus conference [19]. These approaches and other considerations about consensus methods are described in detail in *The Guideline Manual* by NICE [19].

PCOS EBG Example:

All recommendations formulated from each evidence review were reviewed three times to ensure consensus among the guideline development group: 1) a first draft recommendation(s) was suggested by the evidence team and sent to the chair for input; 2) a second draft, formulated by the evidence team and the guideline development group chair, was sent to the guideline development group; 3) the second draft of the recommendation(s) was discussed and revised in the monthly guideline development group meeting; 4) the revised recommendation was revisited and finalised upon consensus using a vote technique within the guideline development group in the following monthly guideline development group meeting.

10. Presentation of the Context and Content of the EBG

It is important that both the EBG and the evidence reviews that underpin the EBG are accessible for those who wish to explore the evidence informing the recommendations and any detail that is unwieldy for inclusion in a 'user friendly' version of the EBG. Ideally, a 'user friendly' version will contain the information that is most useful for efficient on-the-spot decision making.

Using the PCOS EBG example, the 'user friendly' version, in printed form and freely available and accessible online in pdf, contains algorithms, introductory information including the scope and methodology used to develop the EBG; chapters for each set of clinical questions; and future research recommendations.

For each clinical question and subsequent recommendations, the clinical need for the question, the body of evidence and the clinical impact of the recommendations is discussed. Appendices include a list of all EBG committee members, a dissemination plan, glossary and implementation tools.

A larger 800 page supplementary document is freely available and accessible online in pdf which contains all of the evidence reviews that inform the recommendations in the EBG. If the EBG contains technical terms and complicated concepts and technologies not familiar to the general population, translating parts of, or the whole EBG into a consumer friendly version with key messages using minimal jargon has many benefits.

It empowers consumers to make informed health decisions according to their personal needs and preferences [2] and enables shared decision making among clinicians and patients. Algorithms and other supplementary tools that summarise the recommendations and present a clear clinical pathway are invaluable to the usability and uptake of the EBG.

Ideally one page long, they are designed to support quick decision making in the clinical setting [1].

Example PCOS EBG algorithms can be found at: http://www.managingpcos.org.au/pcos-evidence-based-guidelines.

11. Finalising EBG Content and Preparing for Dissemination

Different factors make EBGs differently usable and accessible. The evidence about efficient dissemination strategies is limited [45]. A larger EBGDG may allow for informal dissemination into many different networks, boards, institutions, communities and populations simply by spreading the word.

Endorsement by a guideline development body, whether local, national or international not only extends the dissemination of the EBG but also adds credibility.

An EBG that is available only online will be far less expensive and will reach a larger audience, however the argument may be made that a printed copy may be easier to reach in a clinician's office.

Publicising a guideline in magazines, scientific and medical journals, news reports and internet sites, not only raises awareness about a condition or topic, but also informs consumers about what their clinicians should be doing [2] and alerts the audience who have not yet been reached through other dissemination strategies.

Interestingly, Grol et al. reported that recommendations mentioned in the media or implementation programs were more likely to be used (74%, p=0.06) [46].

The bottom line is that the EBG needs to be identifiable and accessible if it is to be useful.

The hard work, time and expense is largelywasted if EBGis not easily available tothe target audience beyond the initial publicationdate [13].

12. Public Consultation

Aside from consultation and drafting within the committees of the EBG, it is important to test the clarity and usability externally.

The consultation process may be prescribed by the guideline body or the organisation under which the EBG is funded and the most important point is to circulate as widely as possible [1].

It will be easier for both the EBGDG and the external contributor to respond via a form, either online in a survey format or in a document that can be easily emailed or return posted with minimal technology required. While responses to individuals who provide comments is not required, responses to each of the comments and subsequent amendments, after discussion among the EBGDG, should be recorded and be made publicly available.

PCOS EBG Example:

Public and targeted consultation was conducted for a period of 30 days commencing 5th March 2011 in accordance with the legislative requirements set out in section 14A of the *National Health and Medical Research Council Act 1992* as outlined in the NHMRC standards and procedures for externally developed guidelines (2007) [51]. Public consultation was invited via an advertisement in 'The Australian' which directed the reader to content on the Jean Hailes Foundation for Women's Health website and a contact phone number.

The organisations approached for targeted consultation were:

- PCOS Australian Alliance Strategic Advisory Group
- PCOS Australian Alliance members
- Polycystic Ovary Syndrome Association of Australia (peak consumer group)
- Australian Indigenous Doctors Association
- Royal Australian College of General Practitioners
- Royal Australian and New Zealand College of Obstetricians and Gynaecologists
- Royal Australasian College of Physicians
- Endocrine Society of Australia
- Fertility Society of Australia
- Androgen Excess and PCOS Society
- CRANA plus (remote area health professionals)
- Australian Nursing Federation
- Dietetics Association of Australia
- Australian Psychological Society
- PCOS UK (Professor Adam Balen)
- Therapeutic Goods Administration
- Australian Government, Department of Health and Ageing, Pharmaceutical Benefits Branch

Details of submissions arising from public consultation and the response of the guideline development groups as well as how the guidelines were altered as a result of their inclusion are available upon request (jhf.diabetes@monash.edu).

UPDATING

EBGs are reliable because they are based on the best available, most current evidence so to keep up with the most recent research and reflect changes in clinical practice, EBGs need to be revised and updated [1]. Guidance from different bodies suggest revisions anywhere from two to five years and this will likely depend on the profusion and frequency of research published on the topic.

PCOS EBG Example:

The guideline development groups will be re-convened to review relevant sections of this guideline if any of the following occur within five years:

- a change in the indications registered by the Therapeutic Goods Administration for any drug included in this guideline; or
- publication of any new major randomised controlled trials or systematic reviews that potentially have a bearing on the safety of the recommendations in this guideline.

Further detail about the updating process can be found in *The Guideline Manual* by NICE [19].

Conclusion

It is hoped that this chapter provided practical guidance, using an example EBG and direction to practical resources about EBG development. For more detailed guidance on various aspects of EBG development, and for guidance on topics not covered here such as dissemination, implementation and evaluation, the following resources may be helpful:

- Centre for Clinical Effectiveness (CCE). Guideline development toolkit [1].
- Scottish Intercollegiate Guideline Network (SIGN). SIGN 50: A guideline developers' handbook [21].
- National Institute for Health and Clinical Excellence (NICE). The Guideline Manual [19].
- National Health and Medical Research Council (NHMRC) Information for Guideline Developers http://www.nhmrc.gov.au/ guidelines/information-guideline-developers [35]
- National Health and Medical Research Council (NHMRC). Procedures and requirements for meeting the 2011 NHMRC standard for clinical practice guidelines [17]
- New Zealand Guidelines Group (NZGG). Handbook for the Preparation of Explicit Evidence-Based Clinical Practice Guidelines [20].
- The AGREE II Instrument. http://www.agreetrust.org/ [32].

References

[1] Harris C, Turner T, Wilkinson F. Guideline development toolkit. Australia: *Centre for Clinical Effectiveness*, Southern Health, Melbourne 2008.

[2] Woolf S, Grol R, Hutchinson A, Eccles M, Grimshaw J. Clinical guidelines: potential benefits, limitations, and harms of clinical guidelines. *Brit. Med. J.* 1999 Feb 20;318(7182):527-30.

[3] Teede H, Misso M, Deeks A, Moran L, Stuckey B, Wong J, et al. Assessment and management of polycystic ovary syndrome: summary of an evidence-based guideline. *Med. J. Australia.* 2011;195(6):S65-S112.
[4] Turner T, Misso M, Harris C, Green S. Development of evidence-based clinical practice guidelines (CPGs): comparing approaches. *Implement Sci.* 2008;3(45).
[5] Thomson R, Lavender M, Madhok R. Fortnightly review: how to ensure that guidelines are effective. *Brit. Med. J.* 1995 July 22, 1995;311(6999):237-42.
[6] Misso M, Pitt V, Jones K, Barnes H, Piterman L, Green S. Quality and consistency of clinical practice guidelines for diagnosis and management of osteoarthritis of the hip and knee: a descriptive overview of published guidelines. *Med. J. Aust.* 2008;189(7):394-9.
[7] Burgers J, Bailey J, Klazinga N, Van Der Bij A, Grol R, Feder G. Inside guidelines: comparative analysis of recommendations and evidence in diabetes guidelines from 13 countries. *Diabetes Care.* 2002 Nov;25(11):1933-9.
[8] Pencharz J, Grigoriadis E, Jansz G, Bombardier C. A critical appraisal of clinical practice guidelines for the treatment of lower-limb osteoarthritis. *Arthritis Res.* 2002;4(1):36-44.
[9] Poitras S, Avouac J, Rossignol M, Avouac B, Cedraschi C, Nordin M, et al. A critical appraisal of guidelines for the management of knee osteoarthritis using AGREE criteria. *Arthritis Res. Ther.* 2007 Dec 6;9(6):R126.
[10] van Tulder M, Tuut M, Pennick V, Bombardier C, Assendelft W. Quality of primary care guidelines for acute low back pain. *Spine.* 2004 Sep 1;29(17):E357-62.
[11] World Health Organization. Guidelines for WHO Guidelines. Global *Program on Evidence for Health Policy*: World Health Organization 2003.
[12] Zhang W, Moskowitz R, Nuki G, Abramson S, Altman R, Arden N, et al. OARSI recommendations for the management of hip and knee osteoarthritis, part I: critical appraisal of existing treatment guidelines and systematic review of current research evidence. *Osteoarthr Cartilage.* 2007 Sep;15(9):981-1000.
[13] Buchan H, Currie K, Lourey E, Duggan G. Australian clinical practice guidelines--a national study. *Med. J. Aust.* 2010;192(9):490-4.
[14] Alonso C, P, Irfan A, Sola I, Gich I, Delgado-Noguera M, Rigau D, et al. The quality of clinical practice guidelines over the last two decades: a systematic review of guideline appraisal studies. *Qual. Saf. Health Care*. 2010;19(6):1-7.
[15] Grilli R, Magrini N, Penna A, Mura G, Liberati A. Practice guidelines developed by specialty societies: the need for a critical appraisal. *Lancet.* 2000 Jan 8;355(9198):103-6.
[16] March W, Moore V, Willson K, Phillips D, Norman R, Davies M. The prevalence of polycystic ovary syndrome in a community sample assessed under contrasting diagnostic criteria. *Hum. Reprod.* [Research Support, Non-U.S. Gov't]. 2010 Feb;25(2):544-51.
[17] National Health and Medical Research Council. Procedures and requirements for meeting the 2011 NHMRC standard for clinical practice guidelines. NHMRC; 2011.
[18] Council of Europe. *Developing a Methodology for Drawing up Guidelines on Best Medical Practice*. Committee of Ministers of the Council of Europe; 2001.
[19] National Institute for Health and Clinical Excellence. *The Guideline Manual.* NICE; 2007.

[20] New Zealand Guidelines Group. *Handbook for the Preparation of Explicit Evidence-Based Clinical Practice Guidelines*. NZGG; 2001.

[21] Scottish Intercollegiate Guideline Network. SIGN 50: *A guideline developers' handbook*. SIGN; 2004.

[22] Littlejohns P, Cluzeau F, Bale R, Grimshaw J, Feder G, Moran S. The quantity and quality of clinical practice guidelines for the management of depression in primary care in the UK. *Br. J. Gen. Pract.* 1999 Mar;49(440):205-10.

[23] Graham I, Beardall S, Carter A, Glennie J, Hebert P, Tetroe J, et al. What is the quality of drug therapy clinical practice guidelines in Canada? *Can. Med. Assoc. J.* 2001 Jul 24;165(2):157-63.

[24] Shaneyfelt T, Mayo-Smith M, Rothwangl J. Are guidelines following guidelines? The methodological quality of clinical practice guidelines in the peer-reviewed medical literature. *J. Am. Med. Assoc.* 1999 May 26;281(20):1900-5.

[25] Varonen H, Makela M. Practice guidelines in Finland: availability and quality. *Qual. Health Care.* 1997 Jun;6(2):75-9.

[26] Ward J, Grieco V. Why we need guidelines for guidelines: a study of the quality of clinical practice guidelines in Australia. *Med. J. Australia.* 1996 Nov 18;165(10):574-6.

[27] Boluyt N, Lincke C, Offringa M. Quality of evidence-based pediatric guidelines. Pediatrics. 2005 May;115(5):1378-91.

[28] Cates J, Young D, Bowerman D, Porter R. An independent AGREE evaluation of the Occupational Medicine Practice Guidelines. *Spine J.* 2006 Jan-Feb;6(1):72-7.

[29] de Haas E, de Vijlder H, van Reesema W, van Everdingen J, Neumann H. Quality of clinical practice guidelines in dermatological oncology. *J. Eur. Acad. Dermatol. Venereol.* 2007 Oct;21(9):1193-8.

[30] Harpole L, Kelley M, Schreiber G, Toloza E, Kolimaga J, McCrory D. Assessment of the scope and quality of clinical practice guidelines in lung cancer. Chest. 2003 Jan;123(1 Suppl):7S-20S.

[31] Oxman A, Lavis J, Fretheim A. Use of evidence in WHO recommendations. *Lancet.* 2007;369(9576):1883-9.

[32] The AGREE Enterprise. *The Appraisal of Guidelines for Research and Evaluation (AGREE)* Instrument. http://www.agreetrust.org/ (accessed Sep 2011).

[33] Brouwers M, Kho M, Browman G, Burgers J, Cluzeau F, Feder G, et al. AGREE II: advancing guideline development, reporting and evaluation in health care. *Can. Med. Assoc. J.* 2010;182(18):E839-42.

[34] Scott I, Guyatt G. Clinical practice guidelines: the need for greater transparency in formulating recommendations. *Med. J. Aust.* 2011;195(1):29-33.

[35] National Health and Medical Research Council. A guide to the development, implementation and evaluation of clinical practice guidelines. *NHMRC*; 1999.

[36] Schunemann H, Fretheim A, Oxman A. Improving the use of research evidence in guideline development: 13. Applicability, transferability and adaptation. *Health Res. Policy Syst.* 2006;4:25.

[37] The ADAPTE Collaboration. ADAPTE framework. http://www.adapte.org/rubrique/adapte-framework.php (accessed Sep 2011).

[38] Centre for Reviews and Dissemination. Systematic reviews: CRD's guidance for undertaking reviews in health care. CRD, University of York; 2009.

[39] United States National Library of Medicine. Medical subject headings. [cited 2011 October]; Available from: http://www.nlm.nih.gov/mesh/.

[40] Greenhalgh T. How to Read a Paper - The Medline database. *Brit. Med. J.* 1997;315:180-3.

[41] Moher D, Liberati A, Tetzlaff J, Altman D, Group TP. Preferred reporting items for systematic reviews and meta-analyses: the PRISMA statement. *PLoS Med.* 2009;6(6):e1000097.

[42] Centre for Clinical Effectiveness. Critical Appraisal Templates. CCE, *Southern Health*; 2010.

[43] National Health and Medical Research Council. NHMRC additional levels of evidence and grades for recommendations for developers of guidelines. *NHMRC;* 2009.

[44] The Grade Working Group. *Grading the quality of evidence and strength of recommendations.* http://wwwgradeworkinggrouporg (accessed Sept 2011).

[45] Grimshaw JM, Thomas RE, MacLennan G, Fraser C, Ramsay CR, Vale L, et al. Effectiveness and efficiency of guideline dissemination and implementation strategies. *Health Technol. Assess.* 2004 Feb;8(6):iii-iv, 1-72.

[46] Grol R, Dalhuijsen J, Thomas S, Veld C, Rutten G, Mokkink H. Attributes of clinical guidelines that influence use of guidelines in general practice: observational study. *Brit. Med. J.* 1998 Sep 26;317(7162):858-61.

In: Knowledge Transfer: Practices, Types and Challenges ISBN: 978-1-62081-538-0
Editor: Dragan Ilic

Chapter 9

KNOWLEDGE TRANSFER AND PRACTICE FOR CLINICAL SKILLS PERFORMANCE

Stephen Maloney*
Department of Physiotherapy, School of Primary Health,
Monash University, Australia

ABSTRACT

Effective knowledge transfer between researchers, educators, and clinicians is essential for maintaining best practice in the health disciplines. It is the method by which we aim to enhance the health service delivery for our communities. This chapter examines methods of knowledge transfer for supporting health professional clinical performance.

Competent clinical skills are a combination of theoretical knowledge, manual handling, and effective communication, encapsulated in the clinician-client interaction. Training for optimum performance of clinical skills is a complex and enduring task. Health professional education is a continuum, beginning from entry into an undergraduate program, and continues until the health professional leaves their chosen discipline. This chapter focuses on innovative methods utilised within an undergraduate clinical skills program, techniques for supporting transfer of knowledge to a clinical environment, and the continuing education of health professionals. It tackles issues relating to access and utilisation of educational technologies, and facilitation of a successful knowledge transfer culture.

INTRODUCTION

Effective knowledge transfer between researchers, educators, and clinicians is essential for maintaining best practice in the health disciplines. It is the method by which we aim to enhance the health service delivery for our communities [1-3]. This chapter examines methods of knowledge transfer for supporting health professional clinical performance.

* Corresponding author: E-mail: stephen.maloney@monash.edu

"Okay, you, second from the back in the red jumper. Stand up and tell the group what the important theme is from what I have just said. Can't do it? Well pay attention to this lecture, there is going to be a test!" Most clinicians can recall instances of this style of 'teaching by humiliation' so popular in the health disciplines [4], of dry didactic lectures, and fear driven motivations. Health disciplines are in some way unique in that students can assume educational responsibilies immediately following graduation. In the absence of training or exploration of teaching alternatives, the educator often adopts an unfortunate 'master and apprentice' relationship, with the master falling back upon the way in which they were taught, perpetuating poor knowledge transfer practices [4, 5].

Competent clinical skills are a combination of theoretical knowledge, physical handling, and effective communication, encapsulated in the clinician-client interaction. Training for optimum performance of clinical skills is a complex and enduring task. Health professional education is a continuum, beginning from entry into an undergraduate program, and continues until the health professional leaves their chosen discipline.

This chapter focuses on innovative methods utilised within an undergraduate clinical skills program, techniques for supporting transfer of knowledge to a clinical environment, and the continuing education of health professionals. It tackles issues relating to access and utilisation of educational technologies in knowledge transfer, and facilitation of a successful knowledge transfer culture.

There are boundless directions in which any discussion of knowledge transfer techniques could be led. The scenarios and discussion points within this chapter have been selected for their mix of educational theory and practice, their focus on quantitative methodology less frequently explored within educational literature [6], and the generalisability of these techniques and principles in order tofacilitate adaptation to the readers setting.

Supporting Undergraduate Education

Unfortunately there is scant level-one evidence for identifying the most effective knowledge transfer practices for clinical performance [6]. The current literature fails to make head to head comparisons of knowledge transfer methods, matched for duration of content, with known baseline levels and skill-based outcome measures. It typically focuses on a single professional discipline [7] [8] or incorporates non-clinical elements within their outcome measures, such as general knowledge tests or changes in attitude [9]. The vast majority of investigations contrast their interventions against no education, or delayed education [7, 10-19]. At present, the two take home messages from the literature are that plain didactic approaches are typically inferior for producing clinical based learning outcomes in head-to-head comparisons [20], and that alternative teaching methods including small group learning, role-play, video-based or mannequin based simulation, or computer assisted learning (CAL), produce equivalent clinical performance outcomes [20-25]. On a positive note, this leaves a lot of scope for experimentation.

A barrier to developing clinical skills within an undergraduate setting is the overburdened undergraduate curriculum. Any additional time or resources devoted to one particular skill are at the expense of another [26]. Consideration needs to be taken for limited physical resources (space and room bookings) and human resources i.e. cost of tutoring staff. The combination of these factors highlights the need to have effective, but also efficient, learning methods; the best fit between the task, the evidence, and the finite resources available.

The use of Web-based technologies is often heralded as an avenue for enhancing the efficiency in education.This is largely achieved through asynchronous education where the student can access the learning resources at a time when they are most likely to be willing to engage with the material, and by facilitating self-directed learning through sourcing multimedia learning materials [27]. However, it is not without its own inherent challenges. Web-based instruction material often implies the need for a high level of computer literacy from both students and academics. With underperformers typically over-rating their performance [28], methods encouraging self-direction still require provision of learner feedback and clear communication of the expected performance benchmark [29, 30]. Self-video of performance can be a powerful learning tool, facilitating an external view-point for the performer. It has been used for supporting clinical skill development in a variety of health settings including communication skills in medical students [31, 32]. However, coordinating access to central filming equipment creates a new administrative and resource burden.

In exploring the issues surrounding the implementation of technology-based solutions to enable efficient and effective knowledge transfer, it is useful to apply the key points to an existing health professional program, the Monash University Physiotherapy program, Victoria, Australia. A program becoming renowned for its creative educational solutions whilst maintaining strong theoretical underpinning.

The Monash program explored the use of self-video of performance as a tool for providing an external view-point of performance, and as a method of providing evidence of student skill accomplishment before entry into the clinical environment. This is not a new technique, however the challenge was to decentralise the equipment and recording processes, placing the student as producer as well as the performer. The activity was anticipated to supplement 'traditional' practical-room based tutoring, where the students typically receive a demonstration of the skill, participate in clinical reasoning to allow tailoring to different patient contexts, and practice under tutor supervision.

The introduction of this ambitious teaching activity provided an opportunity to explore the different processes taken by staff to maximise the chance of success from a technological standpoint, and in achieving its desired educational objectives. The activity can be summarised by the following required student actions:

- Access a patient scenario that required utilisation of the practical class skill, and consider how the skill may be applied or modified to meet the scenario requirements.
- Film five minutes of footage of themselves as therapists managing the client in the prescribed scenario.
- Upload footage to the Web-based learning system for review by remote tutors who would provide feedback on areas of strength and weakness in the technical, or communication, aspects of the performance.
- View an exemplar peer performance that was selected by the tutor and made available for student viewing via the Web-based system.
- Write a 200-word submission reflecting on their original performance in contrast to the peer-benchmark performance and the tutor's feedback.

Careful planning occurred before the semester began, choosing a weekly skills task that could be recorded with simple footage captured by a single camera view. Written scenarios were then created to allow the student to consider how the skill might be adapted to the individual client, and demonstrated. An example of a patient scenario allocated to students to role-play and apply their skills is as follows:

> "Please submit a 5 minute video that demonstrates a brief 'mobility assessment' on Mr/Mrs Wen, 60yo. Your interview has established he/she is energetic, impulsive and does not have their hearing aids!"

Contemporary university students are generally computer literate and embrace new technology [33], but assuming students possess the skills for completing this task places the activity at risk of being viewed negatively by the students, reducing its chance of success and therefore its potential educational value. A survey of incoming third year students, the cohort in which this teaching and learning activity was to be applied, discovered that approximately 90% of students had ready access to digital filming equipment, in the forms of mobile phones or digital cameras, and that 100% of students were happy to source equipment. To confirm this students were also invited to submit a small segment of digital video 'saying hello' to the unit coordinator as a check of their system.

At the beginning of the semester, students were provided with a training class covering technical aspects of the task submission, including how to submit the electronic files to the universities online learning system, along with explicit descriptions of what would constitute an adequate performance. The students were provided with a list of hints to minimise the risk of technical problems with their submissions including 1) submitting in any file type, 2) utilising any mock-patients i.e. family member or student colleagues, 3) maximising auditory quality by reducing back-ground noise or echo i.e. film in a carpeted room.

From the outline of the above task, it can be seen that the staff increased success of the activity through a number of methods. They pre-warned, and pre-trained the students as to the technological requirements of the task. They provided explicit instruction as to what was expected of the performances. The task provided an external view-point of performance, facilitating the students' ability to self-evaluate their level of competence.

> "I found that converting medical literature into lay terms was difficult; but after watching back my clip, I think I achieved this successfully. Also, my patient (grandmother) found it very difficult to relax during the pendular exercises. I'm not entirely sure if this would be a common occurrence in clinics but found the management of this problematic; I think I may have been perceived as rude…" Segment of de-identified student reflection (May, 2011)

The scenario was designed to be simplistic but to also allow the student to show elements of their clinical reasoning in designing the skill components to be demonstrated. Small group learning and student discussion took place as students informally work-shopped their 'scripts' for the intended performances. There was room for student creativity in the performance itself and in editing the final submission. In addition to self-evaluation, the student was provided with tutor-based feedback, and a peer-benchmark performance as selected by the tutor. Closure on the task was obtained through the brief segment of reflective writing. A de-identified segment of a student's reflection is quoted below, illustrating the relationship between self-assessment and the peer-benchmark.

> "In reflection of my video I found that Mel's [peer-benchmark performance] explanation about the surgery was really good. She was able to explain to the patient very smoothly and in appropriate language what the surgery involved. Whereas in mine I struggled to swap physiotherapy terminology [sic] to lay mans terms, and to flow smoothly through the process, unlike Mel who was able to sequentially inform her patient on what happened. I tended to add too much information or repeat things I had already stated.
>
> Mel's patient rapport with her patient was very natural, though i do think that the rapport i built with my patient was also natural.
>
> I did forget to mention that the pain may still be present after surgery for a little while like Mel did, which would be reassuring for the patient and something to remember for the future.
>
> In comparison to Mel's video I thought that my exercise prescription was really good, and that I covered all areas that are required when giving the patient exercises, like aim, amount, warnings and watching them perform the task." Segment of de-identified student reflection (March, 2011)

The success of this program went beyond the students' enthusiastic uptake and successful completion of the task. The process allowed for decentralisation of the video recording processes and a reduction of the time-pressure of tutors within the practical classes knowing that there were further feedback opportunities. It allowed tutors to notice which aspects of skills were being 'missed' or 'misinterpreted' by the student cohort, providing feedback on the skills teaching, allowing feed-forward to upcoming practical classes. For students it provided a bank of self-performance that could be used for revision, and monitoring change in competence over time.

This knowledge transfer technique was only completed six times across the semester to minimise the burden of the task on student time. It was also limited to selected skills covering the domains of interview, assessment, treatment, and exercise prescription. It was felt that the benefits in attuning the students' self-evaluative ability may positively influence clinical skills not selected for these tasks. A traditional approach may have been more appropriate for skills that students find particularly challenging and/or confusing, that carry high risk of patient harm if completed incorrectly, or where demonstration of the skill is likely to raise questions from the students which are best dealt with in real-time.

Supporting the Transition to Clinical Education

There is always a point within an undergraduate clinical skills program where the performance of skills transitions from practice on simulated patients and student colleagues, to engaging with the real health care consumers within a clinical-setting. This transition from campus-based education to the clinical environment provides the next context for discussing techniques supporting knowledge transfer.

This transition from educational environments brings a number of unique challenges for the student, and for the academic. There is a vast increase in the transactional distance between the university and the student [34], a further shift towards adult learning styles and with it the need to develop as a critically reflective practitioner able to learn from ones mistakes and experiences [35]. The learner must adjust to the diversity of practice techniques specific to the health care setting, or perhaps specific to their particular clinical educator.

From the perspective of the university-based educator, the transition in educational settings raises new challenges in how to facilitate student acquisition of new knowledge, or supported enquiry of existing knowledge and practice. How does an educator overcome the transactional distance? How do they support the equity of learning experiences for a student cohort that is now largely dictated by the patient caseload?

One such method for supporting ongoing 'out of sight' development of clinical skills within a clinical environment is to facilitate the development of critically reflective practitioners. Health practitioners use reflection to analyse and restructure the knowledge that helps them guide their clinical practice [36, 37].

In health professional education, reflective practice is seen as a potential means for facilitating self-improvement from everyday clinical encounters, promoting an up-to-date knowledge base, and enabling life-long learning [38]. Teaching students how to become reflective practitioners has the potential to greatly enhance the theoretical and practical worth of their clinical placements [39].

One validated method for promoting students to be reflective practitioners, are critically reflective essays. Students are graded on their ability to demonstrate learning based on past personal experiences in the clinical setting [40, 41]. Although a number of approaches could be appropriate, the Monash University Physiotherapy program educated the students on a reflective cycle based on the work of Gibbs et al. (1988). The modified Gibbs cycle consists of six stages of reflection 1) the description of the event i.e. what happened, 2) what they were thinking and feeling at the time of the event, 3) an evaluation of what was good and bad about the experience, 4) an analysis of the experience in terms of what sense they can make from it, 5) a conclusion as to what else could have been done, and 6) the development of an action plan should a similar event occur again [42]. Assessment of reflective practice, or reflective writing, is somewhat contentious, however the Monash Program choose to make the essay summative to signify the level of importance of the activity and given that assessment is a driver of learning [43]. The following quotations are taken from a single student's reflective essay to help illustrate the process utilised, and the educational value for developing clinical performance, in this case, relating to an issue with communication within the clinician team:

> "I returned to the PT department and asked two Grade One physiotherapists who had previous experience on the surgical ward, about how to go about the situation. One was too busy, and the other provided me with a referral template which he believed would be suitable….
>
> I returned the following Monday to find 13 messages left from the physiotherapist who received my referral with instructions to return the call immediately. I was then to discover that they were very disappointed with the type of referral they received, as they only accept online referrals via the 'S2S' online system. As a result, no position was available in the knee group for the patient, and they had shredded my referral which they only keep for '24hours.' Consequently, the patients' wife had called to report a complaint about being taken off the waiting list for their preferred outpatient clinic, and thus this reflected poorly not only upon me, but also on the hospital, and upon my supervisor.

> ...I felt confused and annoyed at that point, because I realised that I had attempted to seek help from several others...
>
> ...it made me realise weaknesses in my communication, particularly my ability to assert myself. I realise I should have been more assertive with [supervisor] in voicing what I felt my limits where..."

At the conclusion of the academic semester, after grades had been allocated, students anecdotally reported that reflective essays contained a large portion of fabrication. This was due to the students' perception that essays that appeared more 'insightful' and 'dramatic' had increased chance of obtaining a higher grade from the examiners. Our evaluations also uncovered that although a student may have fabricated the event in which they reflected, they considered the reflection to be honest. Aside from the interesting debate as to whether a students reflection needs to be 'genuine', based on real experiences and honest mental processes, to be educationally beneficial, the Monash team set about evaluating barriers and facilitators to promoting genuine authentic reflection. Academic staff were pleased to see that all the factors identified were able to be influenced by the activities design and implementation. It would be natural to expect that the task parameters i.e. word count, the requirement of referenced literature, and summative nature, would influence inauthentic reflection.Perhaps one of the most surprising influences was that students seemed to be reluctant to write about their own feelings and about negative emotions experienced in the clinical setting, as illustrated in the following quotation from an anonymous student survey of the experience:

> "I found it difficult to write about my emotions in a professional manner, and I didn't feel that some of my feelings were appropriate to be voiced in a university task."

We would therefore make the following recommendations for implementing a critically reflective task, as a summative activity, for developing clinical performance 1) begin the reflective training on campus where the process can be discussed with staff and between students, 2) include in the training particular attention to dealing with and reporting emotions, 3) clearly communicate the process based assessment criteria, not the grandeur of the event within the reflection, 4) encourage students to keep a log/diary of significant events during their clinical placements to assist recall when writing the reflective piece, 5) consideration if the situation allows for the task to be a hurdle (done or not done) as compared to a requiring a grade, and 6) as with all tasks, communicate the relevance of the task for the student as for the healthcare professional, and what this skills looks like when mastered in practice.

Let's now go to the other end of the spectrum, from instilling qualities and abilities within the student, to the supply of fast and efficient learning resources to support knowledge revision and transfer for the student on clinical placement. A relatively new technology being adapted to the tertiary education setting for assisting access and engagement with teaching and learning resources are online repositories. So what is a repository and why is it more efficient than lugging your student lecture and practical notes around?

Electronic repositories allow mass storage, management, search and retrieval of data. In short, it allows you to store all of the teaching resources, including videos, lecture notes, practical support material, in one spot, accessible by students, staff and clinical educators from wherever they can gain Internet access. The key to a repository concept though is the ability to meta-tag items with content description, i.e. where it belongs within a curriculum, to allow efficient retrieval from password protected search engines.

Let's examine the benefits from each stakeholder's perspective for their knowledge and practice requirements, before moving on to the barriers and facilitators to its implementation. We will then conclude by considering some future possibilities for this type of functionality offered by repositories.

From the perspective of a clinical student a well-managed repository of learning resources can assist in efficient tracking of resources to support knowledge revision, and video-based instruction to assist in the revision of patient handling relevant to assessment or treatment techniques. Our evaluations have identified that an electronic repository can increase the time students spend revising, whilst decreasing inefficiencies in finding the intended resource, particularly in sourcing video-based content. Students value a resource bank that is attributable to the University, as a type of filter for content quality given that all resources within the repository have either been constructed by an academic, or sourced by an academic within their program.

From the perspective of the clinical educator, a well managed repository of the students teaching and learning resources can allow the educator to browse the content, creating a greater understanding of the students prior knowledge, and making the statement made by many a student in the face of not knowing an answer "no, we didn't learn that", redundant. The repository also provides an opportunity for the educator to feel a sense of engagement with the university curriculum, and within the Monash University context, is actively invited to suggest or contribute learning resources.

From the perspective of the university-based educator, a single storage and access point to teaching and learning resources enables 'mapping' of the curriculum and the ability to retrieve and review content themes. This facilitates curriculum development. It provides instantaneous updating to resources, improving the currency of resources [44], whereas in the past when practical based DVD's were updated, outdated copies remained in circulation. It also provides a protection for maintaining corporate knowledge in the situation of personnel changes. However, implementation of a repository such as of that described requires a large commitment to change processes from academic staff, information technology support, a significant financial outlay, potential ongoing license fees, training of both staff and students, and consideration of a standard labeling system or metadata schema. In summary, it may not be an option open to all educational institutions, but when effectively constructed and managed, can provide wonderful opportunities for supporting knowledge transfer and practice. An interesting situation has now developed where graduating students are requesting continued access to the universities repository post graduation, as a learning support for ongoing clinical development. Perhaps this is a nice segue to transition into our third knowledge transfer context, the post-graduate environment.

Post-Graduate – Supporting Continued Professional Development

Learning within the health professional disciplines does not stop at graduation. It is a continuous process of updating and refining ones skills from research developments, improving processes, and learning from ones own experiences and the experiences of colleagues. We have discussed the 'beginning' in undergraduate education, the 'transition' as the student moves from campus-based education and skills supervision to the less controlled clinical environment, and now we will explore the post-graduate setting for knowledge transfer techniques supporting clinical performance.

Although post-graduate clinical 'students' may be at a different point within the novice to expert educational continuum, the educational principles remain largely unchanged. Subtle differences between populations may include funding arrangements, and the preference for brief educational packages for clinical skill development in contrast to the expensive and long term commitment of a masters or clinical specialty program [45].

Let's link back to one of our earlier points, that scant evidence exists to suggest that one approach to teaching clinical skills is significantly better than another. A recent study by Maloney et al. (2011), designed two short-courses for the continued professional development of clinical skills of multidisciplinary clinicians', one course developed for live 'face-to-face' delivery, and the other for Web-based delivery [46]. The context of the comparison of knowledge transfer delivery methods was 'exercise prescription for falls prevention'. The study investigated three levels of Kirkpatrick's hierarchy of educational outcomes including attendance, adherence, satisfaction, knowledge, and self-reported change in practice [47]. The delivery methods produced comparable learning outcomes for these investigated outcomes. This study provides evidence that outcomes of Web-based continued professional development are not significantly different to those for face-to-face delivery when applied to an inter-professional audience and a clinical performance subject matter that encompasses a broad range of practical skills including clinical decision making, hands on skills, and high level communication.

So what does this all mean for the educator interested in knowledge transfer and practice for clinical skill development in the health professions? Why evaluate the impact of our knowledge transfer techniques if they are producing equivalent clinical performance outcomes? I would address this by first stating that we have chosen a bias toward quantitative findings within this discussion, and that techniques may vary in the student experience of the education.Attention to the narrative and educational experience of the student is relevant for any educational approach. That despite the 'age' of the research field of knowledge transfer and practice, high quality quantitative studies are relatively new [48, 49], and the literature base will surely develop, continuing to mould what is best practice. With comparable results between delivery methods, practical considerations should arguably drive delivery selection choice. These may preference Web-based techniques in their inherent ability to create a more standardised educational product that is less influenced by the style, experience and knowledge of individual presenters. Web-based methods may afford greater protection against the loss of corporate knowledge with loss of or change in personnel, although use of these methods must be considered in the light of the institutions information technology capabilities and supports. In the presence of quantified comparable outcomes between techniques, alternate measures of comparison should be considered, such as the efficiency of the techniques, including economic analyses, to guide decision makers in educational roles.

A report of the top ten issues facing tertiary education institutions was produced by Deloitte, a Canadian professional services firm, in 2011 [50]. Financial issues and the need for cost-management were listed as the number one issue.

> "As funding dries up, some universities are heading into debt for the first time. This is constraining dollars for classroom delivery and research, creating tension among different departments for scarce financial resources and jeopardizing faculty pay and staff increases."
> *Brian McKenna, page 5 [50].*

The third highest identified priority within the report, was identifying priorities, and warned about making decisions 'in the dark',

> "To succeed into the future, institutions must invest in data mining, financial analysis and IT systems that can help them identify optimal service delivery models and ensure they align to student needs. They must rationalize redundant programs, evaluate the continued relevance of costly ones and ensure their curricula keep pace with market changes."
> *Mark Price, page 13 [50].*

Aside from the financial imperatives, greater efficiency in education techniques creates a number of benefits to both the student and the educators. The student might be able to enjoy increased time to explore new areas of interest, develop specialties, or reflect upon performance, largely prohibited within a modern curriculum [51]. From an educator's perspective, it may produce space to create further educational research and development. I would label investigations of educational efficiency as a future direction in the study of knowledge transfer and practice. Improving efficiency, without jeopardising quality, may prove vital for maintaining a sustainable workforce in a time of an ageing population [52].

Other future directions for research and practice, relating to the topics we have covered in this discussion, are the use of online repositories as a vehicle for sharing resources between teaching departments, and between disciplines. Academia is fascinating in that it is often developed in silos, for example, a medicine department, a physiotherapy department and a department of paramedics and emergency health. Despite students within all of these disciplines needing a concrete knowledge of fracture assessment and management, it is most common that teaching staff within all three departments will need to create and deliver their teaching resources in isolation.

Although the academic institution commonly owns the intellectual property, there are a number of barriers preventing the free exchange of resources between departments. Comparatively, within the realms of 'research' and the scientific community, we encourage peer-review, and yet there are minimal mechanisms for similar peer-review in reference to knowledge transfer resources and practices. Developing these mechanisms holds great promise for improving the quality of the educational resources, for student-centered learning, and potential efficiencies for academic staff and educational institutions.

Conclusion

The breadth of ideas discussed within this chapter highlight the endless range of knowledge transfer and practice techniques that can contribute to supporting clinical performance. Arguably the best techniques utilise an equal blend of creativity, underpinned by sound educational theory, and consideration of practical processes and administration.

Careful design and implementation of any technique should be accompanied by consideration of the best methods for measuring the techniques impact on clinical performance outcomes.

An idea for an innovative solution for addressing modern challenges in knowledge transfer is not enough on its own to grow into a successful new practice. Innovative educational practice requires a supportive organizational knowledge transfer culture. A positive culture is facilitated by recognizing the intertwined relationship between academic staff, administrative staff, clinical educators, and students; taking the time to involve all stakeholders in decisions. New knowledge transfer practices, even those that may act to reduce the eventual workload, will require a temporary increase in effort, and a willingness to change from all involved. Sharing the ownership of change, through wide stakeholder involvement, is a simple but important step to effective implementation.

All institutions with a responsibility for education have an abundance of staff highly dedicated to student knowledge transfer and practice. Educators who are open to questioning techniques, and with the self-assurance to invite peer-review and student appraisal, are the key to improving practice. As an educator and clinician, working daily with just such a team provides an excitement about the future of knowledge transfer and practice for the development of clinical performance.

ACKNOWLEDGMENTS

The author would like to acknowledge the academic and professional staff of Monash University Physiotherapy for their contributions to the development of the knowledge transfer practices discussed within this chapter.

REFERENCES

[1] Davis DA, Thomson MA, Oscman AD, Haynes RB. Changing physician performance: a systematic review of the effect of continuing medical education strategies. *JAMA*. 1995;274:700-5.

[2] Davis DA, Taylor-Vaisey A. Translating guidelines into practice: a systematic review of theoretic concepts, practical experience and research evidence in the adoption of clinical practice guidelines. *CMAJ*. 1997(157):408-16.

[3] Mazmanian PE, Davis DA. Continuing medical education and the physician as a learner: guide to the evidence. *JAMA*. 2002(288):1057-60.

[4] Spencer J. Learning and teaching in the clinical environment. *BMJ*. 2003 Mar 15;326(7389):591-4.

[5] Woolley NN, Jarvis Y. Situated cognition and cognitive apprenticeship: a model for teaching and learning clinical skills in a technologically rich and authentic learning environment. *Nurse Educ. Today*. 2007 Jan;27(1):73-9.

[6] Harden M, Grant J, Buckley G, Hart R. BEME Guide No. 1: Best Evidence Medical Education. *Med. Teach*. 1999;21(6):553-62.

[7] Davis D, O'Brien MA, Freemantle N, Wolf FM, Mazmanian P, Taylor-Vaisey A. Impact of formal continuing medical education: do conferences, workshops, rounds,

and other traditional continuing education activities change physician behavior or health care outcomes? *JAMA*. 1999 Sep 1;282(9):867-74.

[8] Bloom BS. Effects of continuing medical education on improving physician clinical care and patient health: a review of systematic reviews. *Int. J. Technol. Assess. Health Care*. 2005 Summer;21(3):380-5.

[9] Coomarasamy A, Khan KS. What is the evidence that postgraduate teaching in evidence based medicine changes anything? A systematic review. *BMJ*. 2004 Oct 30;329(7473):1017.

[10] Kronz JD, Silberman MA, Allsbrook WC, Epstein JI. A Web-based tutorial improves practicing pathologists' Gleason grading of images of prostate carcinoma specimens obtained by needle biopsy: validation of a new medical education paradigm. *Cancer*. 2000 Oct 15;89(8):1818-23.

[11] Harris JM, Salasche SJ, Harris RB. Can Internet-based continuing medical education improve physicians' skin cancer knowledge and skills? *J. Gen. Intern. Med.* 2001 Jan;16(1):50-6.

[12] Pagnanelli G, Soyer HP, Argenziano G, Talamini R, Barbati R, Bianchi L, et al. Diagnosis of pigmented skin lesions by dermoscopy: Web-based training improves diagnostic performance of non-experts. *Br. J. Dermatol*. 2003 Apr;148(4):698-702.

[13] Curran VR, Hoekman T, Gulliver W, Landells I, Hatcher L. Web-based continuing medical education (I): field test of a hybrid computer-mediated instructional delivery system. *J. Contin. Educ. Health Prof.* 2000 Spring;20(2):97-105.

[14] Curran VR, Hoekman T, Gulliver W, Landells I, Hatcher L. Web-based continuing medical education. (II): Evaluation study of computer-mediated continuing medical education. *J. Contin. Educ. Health Prof.* 2000 Spring;20(2):106-19.

[15] Hinkka H, Kosunen E, Metsanoja R, Lammi UK, Kellokumpu-Lehtinen P. General practitioners' attitudes and ethical decisions in end-of-life care after a year of interactive Internet-based training. *J. Cancer Educ.* 2002 Spring;17(1):12-8.

[16] Harris JM, Jr., Kutob RM, Surprenant ZJ, Maiuro RD, Delate TA. Can Internet-based education improve physician confidence in dealing with domestic violence? *Fam. Med.* 2002 Apr;34(4):287-92.

[17] Kemper KJ, Amata-Kynvi A, Sanghavi D, Whelan JS, Dvorkin L, Woolf A, et al. Randomized trial of an internet curriculum on herbs and other dietary supplements for health care professionals. *Acad. Med.* 2002 Sep;77(9):882-9.

[18] Gerbert B, Bronstone A, Maurer T, Berger T, McPhee SJ, Caspers N. The effectiveness of an Internet-based tutorial in improving primary care physicians' skin cancer triage skills. *J. Cancer Educ.* 2002 Spring;17(1):7-11.

[19] Khatony A, Nayery ND, Ahmadi F, Haghani H, Vehvilainen-Julkunen K. The effectiveness of Web-based and face-to-face continuing education methods on nurses' knowledge about AIDS: a comparative study. *BMC Med. Educ.* 2009;9:41.

[20] Roche AM, Eccleston P, Sanson-Fisher R. Teaching smoking cessation skills to senior medical students: a block-randomized controlled trial of four different approaches. *Prev. Med.* 1996 May-Jun;25(3):251-8.

[21] Birch L, Jones N, Doyle PM, Green P, McLaughlin A, Champney C, et al. Obstetric skills drills: evaluation of teaching methods. *Nurse Educ. Today.* 2007 Nov;27(8): 915-22.

[22] Crofts JF, Bartlett C, Ellis D, Winter C, Donald F, Hunt LP, et al. Patient-actor perception of care: a comparison of obstetric emergency training using manikins and patient-actors. *Qual. Saf. Health Care.* 2008 Feb;17(1):20-4.

[23] Edwards A, Elwyn G, Hood K, Atwell C, Robling M, Houston H, et al. Patient-based outcome results from a cluster randomized trial of shared decision making skill development and use of risk communication aids in general practice. *Fam. Pract.* 2004 Aug;21(4):347-54.

[24] Haak R, Rosenbohm J, Koerfer A, Obliers R, Wicht MJ. The effect of undergraduate education in communication skills: a randomised controlled clinical trial. *Eur. J. Dent. Educ.* 2008 Nov;12(4):213-8.

[25] Robbins AS, Kauss DR, Heinrich R, Abrass I, Dreyer J, Clyman B. Interpersonal skills training: evaluation in an internal medicine residency. *J. Med. Educ.* 1979 Nov;54(11):885-94.

[26] Bordage G. The curriculum: overloaded and too general? *Med. Educ.* 1987 May;21(3):183-8.

[27] King F. A virtual student: Not an ordinary Joe. *The Internet and Higher Education.* 2002;5(2):157-66.

[28] Kruger J, Dunning D. Unskilled and unaware of it: how difficulties in recognizing one's own incompetence lead to inflated self-assessments. *J. Pers. Soc. Psychol.* 1999 Dec;77(6):1121-34.

[29] Palmer P, Henry J, Rohe D. Effect of videotape replay in the quality and accuracy of student self-evaluation. *Physical Therapy.* 1985;65:497-500.

[30] Miller P. Self assessment: the disconnect between research and rhetoric. *Physiotherapy Canada.* 2008(60):117-24.

[31] Lane JL, Gottlieb RP. Improving the interviewing and self-assessment skills of medical students: is it time to readopt videotaping as an educational tool? *Ambul. Pediatr.* 2004 May-Jun;4(3):244-8.

[32] Marteau TM, Humphrey C, Matoon G, Kidd J, Lloyd M, Horder J. Factors influencing the communication skills of first-year clinical medical students. *Med. Educ.* 1991 Mar;25(2):127-34.

[33] Oblinger JL, Pearl DK, Boardman CL, Saqr H, Prior TW, Scheithauer BW, et al. Diagnostic and prognostic value of glycosyltransferase mRNA in glioblastoma multiforme patients. *Neuropathol. Appl. Neurobiol.* 2006 Aug;32(4):410-8.

[34] Garrison R. Theoretical Challenges for Distance Education in the 21st Century: A Shift from Structural to Transactional Issues. *The International Review of Research in Open and Distance Learning.* 2000;1(1):1-20.

[35] Abela J. Adult learning theories and medical education: a review. *Malta Medical Journal.* 2009;21(1):11-8.

[36] Schon D. *The reflective Practitioner.* New York: Basic Books; 1983.

[37] Schon D. *Educating the reflective practitioner.* San Francisco: Jossey Bass; 1987.

[38] Shepard KF, Jensen GM. Physical therapist curricula for the 1990s: educating the reflective practitioner. *Phys. Ther.* 1990 Sep;70(9):566-73; discussion 73-7.

[39] Roche A, Coote S. Focus group study of student physiotherapists' perceptions of reflection. *Medical Education.* 2008;42:1064-70.

[40] Mann K, Gordon J, MacLeod A. Reflection and reflective practice in health professions education: a systematic review. *Adv. Health Sci. Educ. Theory Pract.* 2009 Oct;14(4):595-621.

[41] Plack MM, Driscoll M, Blissett S, McKenna R, Plack TP. A method for assessing reflective journal writing. *J. Allied Health.* 2005 Winter;34(4):199-208.

[42] Gibbs G. Learning by doing: *a guide to teaching and learning methods.* . EMU, editor. UK: Oxford Brookes University; 1988.

[43] Bourner T. Assessing reflective practice. Education and Training. 2003;45(5):267-72.

[44] Grabe M, Christopherson K. Optional student use of online lecture resources: resource preferences, performance and lecture attendance. *Journal of Computer Assisted Learning.* 2008;24(1):1-10.

[45] Gruppen L, Wolf F, Van Voorhees C, Stross J. Information-seeking strategies and differences among primary care physicians. *A Journal for Continuing Education Professionals in Health Sciences.* 1987;7(3):18-26.

[46] Maloney S, Haas R, Keating J, Molloy E, Jolly B, Sims J, et al. The efficacy of Web-based versus face-to-face delivery of falls prevention exercise prescription education to health professionals: a randomised trial. *J. Med. Internet Res.* (forthcoming).

[47] Hutchinson L. Evaluating and researching the effectiveness of educational interventions. *BMJ.* 1999 May 8;318(7193):1267-9.

[48] Chen FM, Bauchner H, Burstin H. A call for outcomes research in medical education. *Acad. Med.* 2004 Oct;79(10):955-60.

[49] Harden RM, Grant J, Buckley G, Hart IR. Best Evidence Medical Education. *Adv. Health Sci. Educ. Theory Pract.* 2000;5(1):71-90.

[50] Deliotte. Making the Grade 2011. *A study of the top 10 issues facing tertiary institutions.* Canada.: Deloitte Touche Tohmatsu Limited. 2011.

[51] Binienda J, Schwartz M. Threading Geriatrics Content through a Four-year Curriculum. *Academic Medicine*:. 2001;76(5):526-7.

[52] Hogan W. Review of Pricing Arrangements in Residential Aged Care, *Aged Care Price Review Taskforce.* Canberra: Australian Government2004.

[53] Boyer EL. Clinical practice as scholarship. *Holist. Nurs. Pract.* 1996 Apr;10(3):1-6.

In: Knowledge Transfer: Practices, Types and Challenges ISBN: 978-1-62081-538-0
Editor: Dragan Ilic

Chapter 10

What Role Can Journal Clubs Play in Knowledge Transfer?

Dragan Ilic*
Department of Epidemiology and Preventive Medicine,
School of Public Health and Preventive Medicine,
Monash University, VIC, Australia

Abstract

Journal clubs have been operating in various formats for over 100 years in the medical field. Journal clubs aim to promote effective knowledge transfer of medical evidence to clinicians and subsequent uptake into the clinical setting. Clinician awareness, agreement, adoption and adherence of evidence may all act as barriers when translating high quality evidence into practice. This chapter will provide a commentary on the use of journal clubs in knowledge transfer and also proposes a method of utilizing journal clubs as complex interventions as a strategy to translate evidence into practice effectively.

Introduction

Journal clubs have been operating for over 100 years in the medical profession, serving as a common meeting to promote discussion amongst clinicians about the medical literature. [1]These journal clubs were introduced in a bid to assist medical practitioners with a means of being up-to-date with the latest medical literature, without needing to subscribe to the growing number of medical journals. [2, 3]More recently journal clubs have been used as a method for teaching the principles of Evidence Based Medicine (EBM), including critical appraisal, biostatistics and research methodology of medical articles. [4, 5]

EBM was developed as a concept to assist clinicians in making medical decisions by integrating their own clinical expertise, with a patient's values and the best available

* Corresponding author: E-mail: dragan.ilic@monash.edu

evidence. [6]The ability to practice according to the principles of EBM requires that the clinician is competent across the following areas;

1) Converting a clinical scenario into an answerable question;
2) Effectively and efficiently searching the medical literature to identify the evidence;
3) Critically appraising the evidence for its validity and applicability;
4) Integrating the critically appraised evidence into the clinical environment; and,
5) Evaluating the success of the EBM process as it relates to the clinical scenario. [7]

It has been estimated that a clinician in general medicine is required to read 19 articles a day, every day of the year to keep up-to-date with the current medical literature. [8] It was also estimated that the same clinician had only one-hour per week to accommodate this reading requirement. [8]Given this unrealistic scenario, the use and dissemination of these EBM skills has become commonplace in current journal clubs [1].

It is accepted that a significant majority of hospitals, both community and university affiliated, contain some form of journal club within their medical and training programs. [3] This breadth of acceptance within the medical community provides great potential for it to be used as an educational format and tool for knowledge transfer.

Barriers and Enablers to Journal Clubs

Many journal clubs begin with great promise, only to fail after a short period of time. This lack of success may be attributed to a variety of factors including time restrictions, lack of goals, interest or participation. [2, 3]Despite these limitations, journal clubs can be an effective method of facilitating knowledge transfer if they are multifaceted in their approach. Factors such as being student/clinician centred, problem based, demonstrate translating theory into practice, interactive and teach lifelong learning skills relevant to the learner's immediate goals or long-term clinical practice all contribute to a successful journal club. [9]

The literature suggests that an ideal journal club does not exist. [9] Rather, the format and the structure of the journal club needs to be styled according the needs of the participants, goals of the journal club and the available resources. A successful journal club must identify key outcomes including specific objectives/goals of the journal club and the best method of implementing the journal club in a clinical environment. Common goals of journal clubs, as identified by medical students, educators and clinicians in order or perceived importance are teaching the principles of evidence based medicine, integrating evidence into practice and keeping abreast of the latest literature. [9] Medical disciplines including internal medicine, general practice and emergency medicine have reported best success at implementing and maintaining journal clubs as part of their teaching curriculum. [2, 10]

It has been suggested that journal clubs work best when sessions are kept to a one-hour time limit, with two to three cases based on real-life clinical problems presented. [10] Factors associated with successful journal club implementation include small group sizes, mandatory attendance and delivered as a supplement to formal teaching on EBM. [10] Journal clubs must also relate the task to the participants' and audiences' clinical environment, whilst also using the time to generate discussion or problem solving on particular aspect (e.g. interpretation of biostatistics or methodology. [9]

Journal Clubs and EBM – The Theoretical Paradox

A systematic review of the literature on journal clubs identified that participation in them can significantly improve clinician clinical education skills, reading habits, time and satisfaction. [11] However, despite its potential, no comparative studies to date have identified any change in clinical behaviour, or evaluation whether the evidence discussed in the journal club has been implemented in clinical practice. [11]Whilst journal clubs have promoted clinicians to refine their critical appraisal skills, it seems that the fourth and fifth steps of the EBM process either are not emphasized or practiced in the journal club environment. Many opponents to EBM will argue that the emphasis is unrealistically placed on gathering and critically appraising the evidence in the journal club environment. [12] Traditionally, the evidence hierarchy in EBM has consisted of placing the systematic review and randomized controlled trial (RCT) at the top of the evidence pyramid, with personal experience, anecdote or a case-scenario placed at the bottom due to the potential inherent biases. [6, 12]

In such scenarios the human aspect (i.e. patient values and a clinician's clinical experience) are somewhat overlooked when conducting a modern journal club. Conversely, the emphasis may disproportionately be placed on the critical appraisal aspects of the journal club, and not the expertise in implementing and evaluating its worth in the clinical context. [13]

To overemphasize the importance of one aspect of EBM over another within the journal club environment would be doing a disservice to patients and clinicians.

> "Without clinical expertise, practice risks becoming tyrannized by evidence, for even excellent external evidence may be inapplicable to, or inappropriate for, an individual patient".[6]
>
> ''Without current best evidence, practice risks becoming rapidly out of date to the detriment of patients". [6]

Recommendations for Establishing and Conducting a Journal Club in a Health Setting

The following structure has been proposed when establishing and sustaining a journal club; [11]

1) Journal Club Attendance

- Members should have a regular meeting time and place, with colleagues who share a similar discipline or clinical interest.

2) Journal Club Purpose

- The overall goal of the journal club should be accepted by all members and reviewed regularly to ensure adherence to it. Each journal club meeting should have its own specific aims i.e. to increase knowledge on a particular topic, improve skills, behaviour change etc.

3) *Journal Club Leader*

- Journal clubs operate effectively if governed by a leader, or chair. Their responsibility is to ensure equitable group involvement and identify relevant topics/articles for discussion. The leader should have well rounded skills in order to guide discussion appropriately e.g. clinical, epidemiological, biostatistical.

4) *Journal Club Articles*

- Relevant case-based articles (i.e. based on the need to acquire evidence for a specific patient) should be chosen, in line with the overarching goals of the journal club. Articles should be circulated to all journal club members at least one-week prior to the meeting to ensure a succinct, quality driven discussion.

5) *Journal Club Effectiveness*

- Established critical appraisal techniques should be agreed upon and used consistently within the journal club. Each journal club session should conclude by putting the article within the clinical context and evaluating its potential impact in translating the evidence into clinical practice.

Adopting these recommendations for establishing and conducting a journal club in a health setting promotes several outcomes.

1) *Professionalism*

It has been suggested that regular participation in journal clubs can be associated with an improvement in the professional behaviour, development, ethics and key learning experiences. [1]

2) *Lifelong Learning*

Participation in the journal club will incorporate both self-directed learning and problem-based learning skills. It also promotes experiential learning, [14] with clinicians moving on from knowing EBM and knowing how to practice EBM, to actually showing and practicing EBM in the clinical context.

3) *Integration of Appropriate Evidence into Clinical Practice*

The knowledge gleaned from journal clubs should incorporate evidence from the best available sources – be it RCTs, cohort studies, case-control studies, case reports or personal experience. Evidence from case reports is commonly the basis on which larger case-control and cohort studies are conducted to investigate risk factors and etiology. This trend to accepting case reports and series has been demonstrated with the establishment of several peer-reviewed journals dedicated to only publishing information from this information source. [15, 16]

UtilizingJournal Clubs in the Quest for Knowledge Transfer

Journal clubs have the potential to serve as a congruent facilitating knowledge transfer from the presenting clinician's clinical example to a larger clinical group who may then draw on the presenting example in future cases (Figure I).

Translating knowledge into practice is a multi-step process, with each step facing a different barrier. [17]Differing models of translating evidence into clinical action have been presented. The four step model suggests that the clinician must be aware, then agree, then adopt and finally adhere to the evidence. [18]The rate of compliance with evidence based recommendations significantly decreases across these four stages due to a variety of barriers knowledge, attitudes, beliefs, time and skills. For example, an investigation of the use of clinicians' vaccine guidelines identified that 90% were aware of the evidence, 67% agreed with it, 46% adopted it, and 35% adhere to the evidence in practice. [18]

A recent model of knowledge transfer suggests a seven stage process of translating evidence into practice consisting of; (i) awareness, (ii) acceptance, (iii) applicability, (iv) availability, (v) acted upon, (vi) agreed to and (vii) adhered to. [17]. Taking into account even an 80% transfer of knowledge across each stage would only provide an uptake of evidence in the clinical setting of 21%. [17]

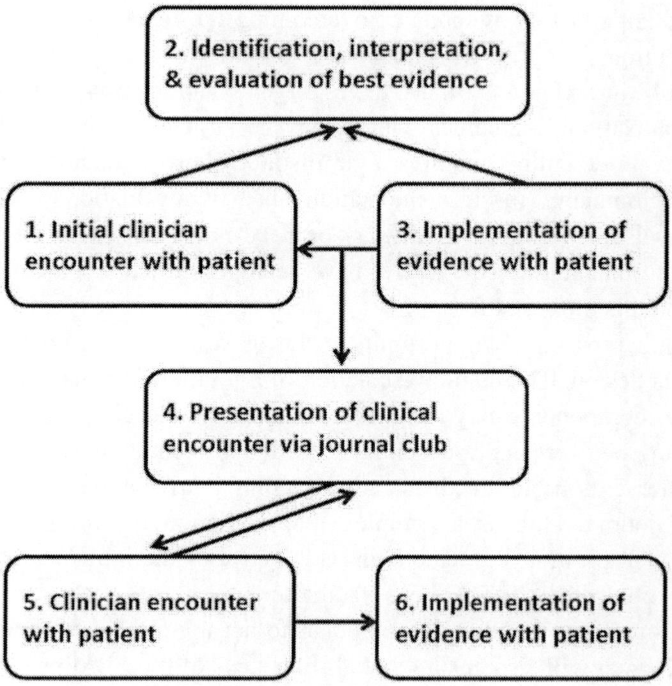

Figure 1.Potential knowledge transfer framework as facilitated by the journal club experience.

Previous research has established that the use of static media such as seminars and lectures are effective at disseminating the evidence, but does not result in the modification of clinician knowledge, attitudes or behaviour with respect to uptake and implementation of evidence in practice. [19, 20].

It has been proposed that a combination of strategies is required if evidence is to be successfully implemented in within the clinical setting. [19, 20]

It has been argued that any such implementation strategy must be tailored to suit the targeted population and issue and should adopt a variety of modalities including; traditional CME seminars, formal conferences and/or workshops, academic detailing, practice based interventions (including clinician and patient education materials), audit with feedback and reminders. [19, 20] These implementation strategies also need to account for non-educational variables that affect clinician behaviour. Evidence is one component however, attitudes and implementation of evidence in the clinical environment is also influenced by the quality of the evidence, characteristics of the clinician, the practice setting and patient factors[20].

The journal club is uniquely positioned to potentially act as a de facto complex intervention that promotes behaviour change with respect to the best evidence (Figure II).

The EBM framework suggests a five step process whereby a clinical problem may be answered by identifying the question, sourcing the literature, critically appraising the evidence, implementing it in practice then evaluating its effectiveness.

The use of journal clubs can facilitate the first three steps of this process – however there may be as much as seven barriers to the uptake of evidence in practice. It can be argued that knowledge presented in the journal club can overcome the first barrier of awareness – since all participants in a journal club will become aware of the evidence and subsequently have new or updated knowledge on the topic. The issue then shifts to the remaining six barriers – from acceptance to adherence in the clinical environment.

There are potentially two methods of overcoming the remaining barriers; (i) the use of complex interventions, or (ii) a refined use of the journal club approach. Complex interventions are interventions that have several interacting components targeting behavioural, organizational outcomes, which may be targeted in their implementation. [21] Using a complex intervention requires four distinct phases including; (i) feasibility and piloting, (ii) development, (iii) implementation and (iv) evaluation. [21]The journal club presents as a novel intervention, which may be used potentially as a complex intervention within itself. No formal studies (i.e. RCTs) have been performed to evaluate the potential use of journal clubs in this proposed format.

A journal club presents an opportunity to be used as a dissemination strategy that is multifaceted in its design. The main presentation of a journal club may be didactic in nature, however the other components may incorporate a number of teaching and knowledge transfer strategies including peer-to-peer counseling, modified academic detailing, implementation of practice based interventions and feedback at proceeding journal clubs.

Trialing the journal club as a complex intervention may promote acceptance of the evidence, which will promote agreement and adherence of its implementation in the clinical environment by clinicians. These steps facilitate a clinician's ability to implement the evidence, which only requires then the clinician to act upon the evidence when applicable. Utilizing this approach will also ensure that all five steps of the EBM process are undertaken, with particular emphasis on the implementation and evaluation of evidence steps in proceeding journal clubs.

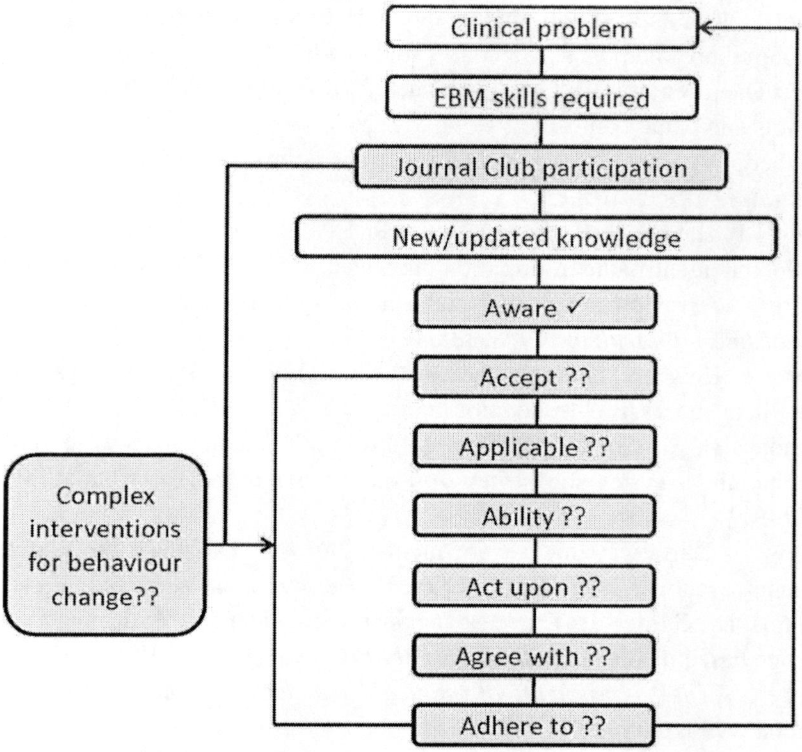

Figure 2. Proposed framework for behaviour change and uptake of evidence into practice using the journal club as a complex intervention.

Conclusion

Currently journal clubs play an important role in the medical community of drawing together clinicians and facilitating knowledge transfer. However, their worth at promoting knowledge transfer and facilitating behaviour change is underutilized. Journal clubs need to be established using a robust framework that can promote active learning within the group setting but more so promote lifelong learning skills to individual clinicians whilst also providing a process in which evidence may be translated into the clinical setting with minimal obstacles preventing optimal patient outcomes.

References

[1] Cave M, Clandin J: Revisiting the journal club. *Medical Teacher* 2007, 29:365-370.

[2] Heiligman R: Resident evaluation of a family practice journal club.*Family Medicine* 1991, 23:152-153.

[3] Linzer M: The journal club and medical education: over one hundred years of unrecorded history.*Postgraduate Medical Journal* 1987, 63:475-478.

[4] Kitching A: Resuscitating the cardiology journal club.*Canadian Journal of Cardiology* 1992, 8:520-522.

[5] Cramer S, Mahoney M: Introducing evidence based medicine to the journal club, using a structured pre and post test: a cohort study.*BMC Medical Education* 2001, 1:6.

[6] Sackett D, Rosenberg W, Gray J, Haynes R, Richardson W: Evidence based medicine: what it is and what it isn't.*BMJ* 1996, 312:71-72.

[7] Rosenberg W, Donald A: Evidence based medicine: an approach to clinical problem-solving.*BMJ* 1995, 310:1122-1126.

[8] Davidoff F, Haynes B, Sackett D, Smith R: Evidence-based medicine: a new journal to help doctors identify the information they need.*BMJ* 1995, 310:1085-1086.

[9] Alguire P: A review of journal clubs in postgraduate medical education.*Journal of General Internal Medicine* 1998, 13:347-353.

[10] Sidorov I: How are internal medicine residency journal clubs organized, and what makes them successful?*Archives of Internal Medicine* 1995, 155:1193-1997.

[11] Deenadayalan Y, Grimmer-Somers K, Prior M, Kumar S: How to run an effective journal club: a systematic review.*Journal of Evaluation in Clinical Practice* 2008, 14:898-911.

[12] Roberts G: Narratives and severe mental illness: what place do stories have in an evidence-based world?*Advances in Psychiatric Treatment* 2000, 6:432-441.

[13] Williams D, Garner J: The case against the evidence: a different perspective on evidence based medicine.*British Journal of Psychiatry* 2002, 180:8-12.

[14] Miller G: *The assessment of clinical skills*/competence/performance. *Academic Medicine* 1990, 65:S63-67.

[15] BMJ: *BMJ Case reports*. Accessed 10/10/2011; Available at; http://casereports.bmj.com.

[16] Kidd M: *Journal of Medical Case Reports*. Accessed 10/10/2011; Available at; http://www.jmedicalcasereports.com.

[17] Glasziou P, Haynes R: The paths from research to improved health outcome.*EBM* 2005, 10:4-7.

[18] Pathman D, Konrad T, Freed G, Freeman V, Koch G: The awareness-to-adherence model of the steps to clinical guidelines compliance. The case of pediatric vaccine recommendations.*Medical Care* 1996, 34:873-889.

[19] Grimshaw J, Eccles M: Is evidence-based implementation of evidence-based care possible?*MJA* 2004, 1810:S50-51.

[20] Davis D, O'Brien M, Freemantle N, Wolf F, Mazmanian P, Taylor-Vaisey A: Impact of formal continuing medical education: do conferences, workshops, rounds, and other traditional continuing education activities change physician behavior or health care outcomes?*JAMA* 1999, 282:867-874.

[21] Craig P, Pieppe P, Macintyre S, Nazareth I, Petticrew M: Developing and evaluating complex interventions: the new Medical Research Council guidance.*BMJ* 2008, 337:a1655.

INDEX

C

D

E

F

G

H

I

J

K

L

M

N

O

P

Q

R

S

T

U

V

W

Y

Z